Diabetic Foot

Martina Zavacká

Diabetic Foot

A Vascular Surgeon's Perspective

nova
science publishers
New York

Library of Congress Cataloging-in-Publication Data

Print ISBN: 979-8-89113-019-7
PDF ISBN: 979-8-89113-065-4
ePUB ISBN: 979-8-89113-159-0

Published by Nova Science Publishers, Inc. † New York

Contents

About the Editor

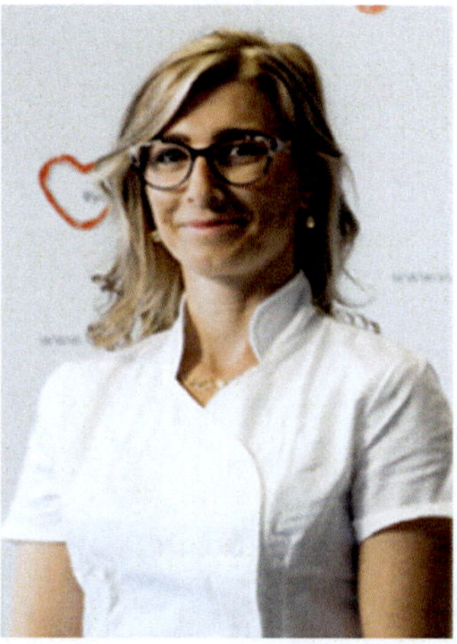

Associate Professor **Martina Zavacká,** MD, Ph.D., MPH

Department of Vascular Surgery, East Slovak Institute of Cardiovascular Diseases, Faculty of Medicine, Pavol Jozef Šafárik University in Košice, Slovakia

Associate Professor Martina Zavacká, MD, Ph.D., MPH is the head of the Department of Vascular Surgery, Faculty of Medicine UPJŠ (LF UPJŠ) and East Slovak Institute for Cardiovascular Diseases (VÚSCH, a.s.). After graduating from LF UPJŠ in Košice, she worked as a Ph.D. student at the 1st Surgical Clinic of the Faculty of Medicine UPJŠ and UNLP, later at the Department of Vascular Surgery Faculty of Medicine UPJŠ and VÚSCH. After successfully passing her dissertation defense, she was awarded a Ph.D. title and continued to work at the Department of Vascular Surgery as a doctor. She became a certified specialist in the field of surgery and vascular surgery. She successfully completed her specialization studies at SMU in Bratislava in the specialization field of Public Health Management Specialist, Master of Public Health (MPH). After a successful habilitation, she was awarded the scientific-pedagogical title of associate professor. She performs pedagogical activities: conducts lectures and practical exercises for students of general and dental medicine in Slovak and English languages. She is a trainer and opponent of several diploma theses, a member of examination commissions for state final examinations in the subject of surgery, and a member of the teaching staff and of the examination commission for specialized examinations in vascular surgery. She is the author and co-author of more than 50 scientific and more than 40 professional publications published in domestic and foreign journals, textbooks, books, and monographs.

Introduction

Martina Zavacká

Diabetic foot patients are among the most complex and most vulnerable of all patient populations.

Diabetic foot syndrome (DFS) is one of the most common late complications of diabetes, significantly affecting patients' quality of life. The WHO defines it as an infection, ulceration, or destruction of the deep tissues of the leg associated with neurological abnormalities and varying degrees of ischemic disease of the lower limbs.

The etiology of diabetic foot ulcers is complex due to their multifactorial nature; polyneuropathy is essential in the pathophysiology of diabetic foot ulceration. The most significant proven risk factors for ulcerations include neuropathy (sensorimotor, autonomic), angiopathy (macro- and microvascular), and increased foot plantar pressure. External factors such as trauma, inappropriate shoes, and infection are also responsible for ulcerations. We must not forget the influence of smoking, poorly compensated diabetes, and other factors affecting the formation of neuropathy and ischemia.

The management of diabetic foot ulcers requires the interdisciplinary collaboration of various medical disciplines and active exchange between physicians and nurses/assistants. The prevalence of DFS is 4% to 15%. DFS is the main reason for the hospitalization of patients among all possible complications of type 2 diabetes. Compared to non-diabetics, the need for above-knee amputation is about 30 to 40 times more increased in patients with type 2 diabetes mellitus. Five-year mortality after amputation is estimated at 39%-68%. It has been found that at least three-quarters of diabetes-related lower limb amputations could have been avoided with proper prevention. It is recommended to protect the feet with suitable, comfortable shoes, preferably shoes indicated for diabetics. It is crucial to avoid exposure to heat (electric pillows, warm baths, etc.) and to dry your feet well after bathing, including between the toes. Care should also be taken when cutting the nails because even a minor injury can form an ulcer. The patient should refrain from smoking and should remember skin care. Using the proper preparations, it is possible to increase the resistance of the skin of the feet and strengthen its natural protective barrier. Adequate adherence to standard treatment strategies and interdisciplinary collaboration can reduce the high number of major amputations. Specialized clinics for the diabetic foot in the 21st century should be multidisciplinary and equipped to coordinate diagnosis, interpretation, and preventive care; perform revascularization procedures; aggressively treat infections; and manage medical comorbidities. The development of distal revascularization techniques to restore pulsatile blood flow to the leg has significantly improved limb salvage. The history of the team approach to treating the diabetic foot records the emergence of a new health profession – podiatric medicine and surgery- and the emergence of the specialties of vascular surgery and wound healing. The partnership of diabetologists, vascular surgeons, and podiatrists can be seen as natural; their skills and knowledge complement one another and lead to more successful limb salvage and functional results.

This book was translated by Dr. Peter Protivňak.

Chapter 1

Anatomy of the Vessels of the Lower Limbs

Lukáš Vaško, MD*

Department of Vascular Surgery, East Slovak Institute of Cardiovascular Diseases, Faculty of Medicine, Pavol Jozef Šafárik University in Košice, Slovakia

Abstract

This chapter describes the anatomy of arteries and veins of the lower limbs.

Key Words: anatomy, veins, arteries, lower limb, abdominal aorta, superficial veins, deep veins

Abdominal aorta and arteries of lower limbs

Abdominal aorta (Pars abdominalis aortae)

The abdominal aorta begins at the diaphragmatic hiatus and runs to the level of the L4 lumbar vertebra. At the level of the L4 vertebra, the abdominal aorta bifurcates into the terminal branches. The abdominal aorta nourishes the organs in the peritoneal cavity; in the region of the retroperitoneum and pelvis, it nourishes a part of the abdominal and pelvic wall and the lower limbs.

From the abdominal aorta branch off:

a, parietal branches: inferior phrenic arteries *(aa. phrenicae inferiores*) and lumbar arteries *(aa. lumbales)*

b, visceral branches:

* Corresponding Author's Email: lvasko@vusch.sk

In: Diabetic Foot
Editor: Martina Zavacká
ISBN: 979-8-89113-019-7

- paired branches: the middle suprarenal arteries *(aa. suprarenales mediae),* renal arteries *(aa. renales),* testicular / ovarian arteries *(aa. testiculares/aa. ovaricae)*
- unpaired branches: celiac trunk *(truncus celiacus*), superior mesenteric artery (*a. mesenterica superior*), inferior mesenteric artery *(a. mesenterica inferior)*

The Celiac trunk *(Truncus coeliacus)* is divided into three branches: the left gastric artery (*a. gastrica sinistra*), common hepatic artery (a. hepatica communis), and splenic artery *(a. splenica).*

Superior mesenteric artery *(a.mesenterica superior)* branches off from the aorta at the level of the L1 and nourishes the loops of the small intestine, duodenum, pancreas, cecum, ascending, and transverse colon.

The branches of the superior mesenteric artery are the following:

- inferior pancreaticoduodenal artery (*a. pancreaticoduodenalis inferior)*
- jejunal and ileal arteries (*aa. jejunales and aa. ileales)*
- ileocolic artery (*a. ileocolica)*
- right colic artery (*a. colica dextra)*
- right flexural artery (*a. flexurae dextrae)*
- middle colic artery (*a. colica media)*

Inferior mesenteric artery *(a.mesenterica inferior)* branches at the L2/ L4-lumbar vertebra level. It goes into the left iliac fossa. It nourishes the descending and ace-shaped part of the large intestine and the rectum. Its branches are the following:

- left colic artery (*a. colica sinistra)*
- sigmoid arteries (*aa. sigmoideae)*
- superior rectal artery (*a. rectalis superior)*

Common iliac artery (a.iliaca communis)

The *pars abdominalis aortae* divides at the level of the L4 vertebra into right and left iliac arteries *(a. iliaca communis dextra and a. iliaca sinistra).*

Internal iliac artery (a.iliaca interna)

The internal iliac artery forms a relatively short trunk. Posterior trunk branches are: iliolumbar lateral sacral, superior gluteal and inferior gluteal arteries (a.*iliolumbalis*, *aa. sacrales laterales*, *a. glutea superior* and *a. glutea inferior*).

The anterior trunk arteries are:

- inferior vesical artery (*a. vesicalis inferior)*
- uterine artery (*a. uterina)* /deferential artery *(a. ductus deferentis)*
- vaginal artery *(a. vaginalis)*
- middle rectal artery (*a. rectalis media),*
- internal pudendal artery (*a. pudenda interna),*
- obturator artery (*a. obturatoria)* passes through the obturator canal *(canalis obturatorius)*

External iliac artery (a. iliaca externa)

The external iliac artery is a relatively thick branch that descends along with the vein of the same name below the inguinal ligament to lacuna vasorum, where it turns into the femoral artery *(a. femoralis*). The external iliac artery sends branches to the anterior abdominal wall muscles. The most important is the inferior epigastric artery (*a. epigastrica inferior).*

- The inferior epigastric artery ascends to the inner surface of the rectus abdominis muscle. It branches out in the rectus abdominis muscle and connects with the superior epigastric artery/internal thoracic artery *(a. epigastrica superior/a. thoracica interna).*

Arteries of the lower limbs

The arteries of the lower limb are branches of the external iliac artery. The main artery is the femoral artery, which enters between the thigh muscles and the popliteal fossa. There it is denoted as the popliteal artery. The popliteal artery splits into a. tibialis anterior and a. tibialis posterior, which nourish the lower leg and gradually branch to a. dorsum et a. planta pedis.

Femoral artery

The femoral artery begins below the inguinal ligament. On the front surface of the thigh, the artery lies in the fossa iliopectinea, where the vein of the same name (*v. femoralis*) runs on the inner side, and the outer side runs the femoral nerve (n. femoralis). From the fossa iliopectinea, the artery descends through the cannalis adductorius into the popliteal fossa.

Femoral artery branches:

- *a. epigastrica superficialis* and *a. circumflexa ilium superficialis*,
- towards the external genitalia: *aa. pudendae externae* (a. *pudenda externa, superficialis et profunda),*
- towards the thigh muscles *a. profunda femoris*, the strongest branch that nourishes most of the thigh muscles. Typically it sends three arteries – *aa. perforantes (prima, secunda, et tertia)* to the flexors of the knee joint.
- in addition, its branch - *a. circumflexa femoris lateralis*- nourishes *the caput et collum femoris,*
- towards the knee joint*:* *a. descendens genus*, which unfolds in the canalis adductorius and accompanies the saphenous nerve

Popliteal artery

The popliteal artery is a direct continuation of the femoral artery. It starts at the distal edge of the cannalis adductorius and ends at the lower edge of the popliteal muscle.

The popliteal artery nourishes the knee joint, to which it sends five branches:

- *a. superior lateralis genus* and *a. superior medialis genus,*
- *a. media genus,*
- *a. inferior lateralis genus,* and *a. inferior medialis genus.*

These arteries create a rich arterial network - *rete articulare genus* and a separate network - *rete patellare* around the patella and *aa. surales* – they branch to the calf muscles.

Anterior tibial artery

The artery begins at the lower edge of the popliteal muscle, passes through the interosseous membrane, and reaches the front side of the foreleg. *A. tibialis anterior* reaches the lower edge of the *retinaculum mm. extensorum,* from where the dorsalis pedis artery continues.

Anterior tibial artery branches into:

- *a. malleolaris anterior lateralis*
  and *a. malleolaris anterior medialis.*

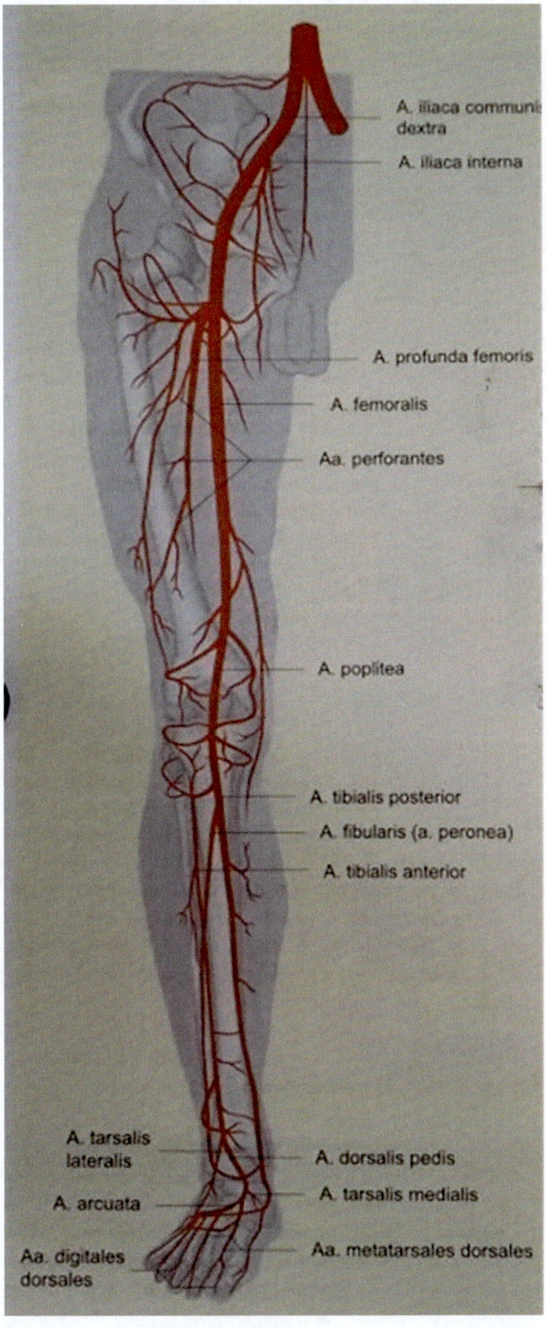

Figure 1.1 Arteriae membri interioris (source: Department of Vascular Surgery VUSCH).

Arteria dorsalis pedis

It runs as a direct continuation of *a. tibialis anterior* on the back of the leg. Underneath the tendon of *m. extensor hallucis longus* and *retinaculus mm. extensorum* and is placed laterally from the tendon of *m. extensor hallucis longus.*

It is also tangible in this space.

Arteria dorsalis pedis gives off:

- *a. tarsea lateralis* and *aa. tarseae mediales*
- *a. arcuata*- four arteries are divided from it – *aa. metetarsales dorsalis,* and each is divided into two arteries- *aa. digitales dorsales*
- *a. plantaris profunda* is a separate strong branch - it continues to the foot, where it joins the *arcus plantaris profundus*

Posterior tibial artery

It is a continuation of the popliteal artery. It runs under the arcus tendinous of the soleus muscle and winds between the superficial and deep groups of calf muscles to the inner ankle.

Branches of the posterior tibial artery:

- *r. circumflexus,*
- *rr. malleolares mediales,*
- *a. fibularis (a. peronea)* - sends *rr. malleolares laterales* and; and gives off *rr.calcanei* to rete calcaneum. The end section of the artery connects to the anterior tibial artery on the back of the leg. In addition, it sends the connecting branch (*r. communicans*) to *a. tibialis posterior* on the calf. By this interconnection, *a. fibularis* creates important collateral circulation.

The posterior tibial artery divides into two arteries:

- *a. plantaris medialis,.*
- *a. plantaris lateralis*, which bends in an arc and connects with *a. plantaris profunda (a. dorsalis pedis*), so that they create a deep arc-shaped connection - *arcus plantaris profundus. Aa. metatarsales plantares* emerge from the arc and continue for a short section as *aa. digitales plantares communes* and end by branching to *aa. digitales plantares propriae* for the adjacent sides of the toes.

Veins of the lower limbs

We divide the veins of the lower limb into two venous systems – the superficial veins (*venae superficiales membri inferioris*) and the deep veins (*venae profundae membri inferioris).*

Venae profundae membri inferioris accompany the arteries of the same name and have the same name. On the foreleg and leg, the deep veins are usually doubled; in the region of the popliteal fossa and on the thigh (*v. poplitea, v. femoralis*), they are single. The deep veins of the lower limb drain most of the blood from the lower limb. They have well-developed venous valves. They are interconnected, and by transaxial connections, they are connected with superficial veins.

Venae superficiales membri inferioris

The superficial veins of the lower limb arise on the planta pedis and dorsum pedis, where they form venous networks - *rete venosum dorsale pedis* and *rete venosum plantare.* The more prominent of the two networks mentioned is the one on the dorsum pedis. *Vv digitales dorsales pedis* are formed from it, which join into *vv. metatarsales dorsales*, which are transversely connected and form the arcus venosus dorsalis pedis.

In a similar way, vv. digitales plantares are formed on the planta pedis, which continue as vv. metetarsales plantares. The arcus venosus plantaris is formed on foot. Both networks of veins are interconnected by veins running in the intermetatarsal spaces on the sides of the leg, where v.marginalis lateralis and v. marginalis medialis are formed.

Great saphenous vein (vena saphena magna)

It begins on the medial edge of the surface of the leg, from where it continues to the inner ankle. After the shin, it emerges along the ventromedial surface accompanied by the saphenous nerve. It continues along the ventromedial surface of the thigh to the saphenous hiatus—the hiatus saphenus projects into the region of the fossa iliopectinea. The great saphenous vein goes deep and ends in the femoral vein. In this area, it receives tributaries:

- from the medial and dorsal surface of the thigh: *v. saphena accessoria,*
- from the lower abdomen and the lateral area of the thigh: *v. epigastrica superficialis, v. circumflexa ilium superficialis,*
- from the external genitalia: *vv. pudendae externae, vv. dorsales superficiales clitoridis (penis), vv. labiales (scrotales) anteriores.*

Small saphenous vein (vena saphena parva)

It is formed on the lateral edge of the leg from the rete venosum dorsale pedis. It continues behind the inner ankle and up the posterior surface of the foreleg to the popliteal fossa. At first, it runs suprafascially, then between two sheets

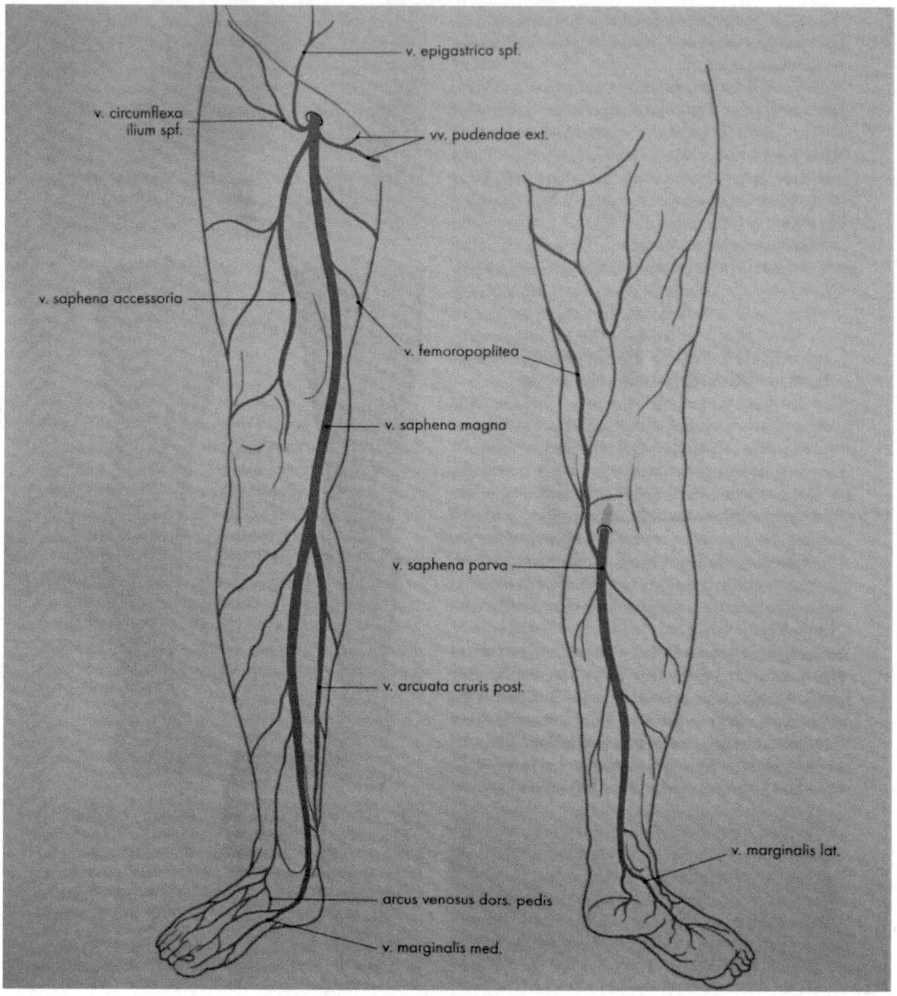

Figure 1.2 Superficial veins of the lower limb (source: Department of Vascular Surgery VUSCH).

of popliteal fascia between the medial and lateral head of the gastrocnemius muscle. It penetrates the popliteal fascia in the popliteal fossa, and flows into the popliteal vein. The popliteal vein is located below the tibial nerve in the middle part of the popliteal fossa. The small saphenous vein collects blood from the lateral area of the back of the leg, the lateral and dorsal surface of the lower leg, and connects with the accessory veins from the back surface of the thigh. The superficial veins of the lower limb form numerous connections with the deep venous system. These important conjunctions, especially with the great saphenous vein, are denoted vv. perforantes (perforators - transfascial connectors). Three vv. perforantes connect the superficial venous system with vv. tibiales posteriores. Venae perforantes, thanks to the valves, regulate the blood flow from the superficial venous networks to the posterior tibial vein. In the case of insufficiency of these valves, the blood flow is reversed into the superficial veins.

References

Borovanský L: Anatomie, Prague, 1978
Čihák R: Anatomy, Galen, 2008

Chapter 2

Diabetes Mellitus from the Surgeon's Perspective

Martina Zavacká, MD*
Department of Vascular Surgery, East Slovak Institute of Cardiovascular Diseases, Faculty of Medicine, Pavol Jozef Šafárik University in Košice, Slovakia

Abstract

Several pathogenic processes are involved in the development of diabetes. It is characterized by hyperglycemia, which arises from disorders of insulin secretion, insulin action, or both causes simultaneously. Symptoms of severe hyperglycemia include polyuria, polydipsia, weight loss, sometimes polyphagia, and blurred vision. Chronic hyperglycemia can also be accompanied by impaired growth and susceptibility to certain infections. Acute, life-threatening consequences of uncontrolled diabetes are hyperglycemia with ketoacidosis or nonketotic hyperosmolar syndrome. Long-term complications of diabetes include retinopathy; nephropathy; peripheral neuropathy with risk of leg ulcers, amputations, and Charcot's joints; autonomic neuropathy causing gastrointestinal, genitourinary, and cardiovascular symptoms, and sexual dysfunction.

Key Words: diabetes mellitus, hyperglycemia, ulcer, amputation, neuropathy, Charcot's joints

General View of Diabetes Mellitus

Diabetes mellitus is a group of metabolic diseases characterized by hyperglycemia, which occurs due to disorders of insulin secretion, insulin action, or

* Corresponding Author's Email: martina.zavacka@upjs.sk

In: Diabetic Foot
Editor: Martina Zavacká
ISBN: 979-8-89113-019-7

both causes simultaneously. Chronic hyperglycemia is associated with long-term damage, dysfunction, and failure of various organs, especially the eyes, kidneys, nerves, heart, and blood vessels.

Several pathogenic processes are involved in the development of diabetes. These range from autoimmune destruction of pancreatic β-cells with subsequent insulin deficiency to abnormalities that lead to insulin resistance. The basis of the abnormalities in the metabolism of carbohydrates, fats, and proteins in diabetes is insufficient insulin action on the target tissues. Insufficient insulin action results from inadequate insulin secretion and/or reduced tissue response to insulin at one or more points in the complex pathways of hormonal activity. Impaired insulin secretion and defects in insulin action often co-occur in the same patient, and it is often unclear which abnormality is the primary cause of hyperglycemia.

Symptoms of severe hyperglycemia include polyuria, polydipsia, weight loss, sometimes polyphagia, and blurred vision. Chronic hyperglycemia can also be accompanied by impaired growth and susceptibility to certain infections. Acute, life-threatening consequences of uncontrolled diabetes are hyperglycemia with ketoacidosis or nonketotic hyperosmolar syndrome.

Long-term complications of diabetes include retinopathy with potential vision loss; nephropathy leading to kidney failure; peripheral neuropathy with risk of leg ulcers, amputations, and Charcot's joints; and autonomic neuropathy causing gastrointestinal, genitourinary, and cardiovascular symptoms and sexual dysfunction. Patients with diabetes have an increased incidence of atherosclerotic cardiovascular, peripheral arterial, and cerebrovascular diseases. Hypertension and abnormalities of lipoprotein metabolism frequently occur in people with diabetes.

The vast majority of diabetes cases fall into two broad etiopathogenetic categories. In the first category - type 1 diabetes, the cause is the absolute lack of insulin secretion. Individuals at increased risk of developing this type of diabetes can often be identified by serological evidence of an autoimmune pathological process occurring in the pancreatic islets and by genetic markers. In the second, much more general category, type 2 diabetes, the cause is a combination of resistance to the action of insulin and an insufficient compensatory response of insulin secretion. In this second category, hyperglycemia may be sufficient to cause pathological and functional changes in various target tissues. Still, it may be present for a long time before the diagnosis of diabetes without clinical symptoms.

The degree of hyperglycemia can change over time depending on the extent of the underlying disease process. A disease process may be present but not advanced enough to cause hyperglycemia. The same disease process can cause impaired fasting glycemia (IFG) and/or impaired glucose tolerance (IGT) without meeting the criteria for a diagnosis of diabetes. In some individuals with diabetes, adequate glycemic control can be achieved with weight reduction, exercise, and/or oral agents. These individuals, therefore, do not need insulin. Other individuals have some residual insulin secretion and require exogenous insulin for adequate glycemic control, but they can survive without it. Individuals with extensive β-cell destruction and thus no residual insulin secretion need insulin for survival.

Type 1 diabetes (destruction of β-cells that usually leads to absolute insulin deficiency) Immune-mediated diabetes mellitus

This form of diabetes, which accounts for only 5–10% of diabetic patients, previously referred to as insulin-dependent or juvenile-onset diabetes, results from cell-mediated autoimmune destruction of pancreatic β-cells. Markers of β-cell immune destruction include islet cell autoantibodies, insulin autoantibodies, GAD autoantibodies (GAD65), and autoantibodies to tyrosine phosphatases IA-2 and IA-2p. The disease also has strong HLA associations linked to the DQA and DQB genes and is influenced by the DRB genes. These HLA-DR/DQ alleles can be predisposing or protective.

In this form of diabetes, the rate of β-cell destruction is highly variable, being fast in some individuals (mainly infants and children) and slow in others (especially adults). Some patients, especially children and adolescents, may have ketoacidosis as the first manifestation of the disease. Others have mild fasting hyperglycemia that can rapidly turn into severe hyperglycemia and/or ketoacidosis in the presence of infection or other stress. Others, especially adults, may retain residual β-cell function sufficient to prevent ketoacidosis for many years; such individuals eventually become insulin dependent for survival and are at risk for ketoacidosis. There is little or no insulin secretion in this late stage of the disease, as indicated by low or undetectable plasma C-peptide levels.

Autoimmune β-cell destruction has multiple genetic predispositions and is also related to environmental factors that are still poorly defined. Although patients with this type of diabetes are rarely obese, obesity is not incompatible with the diagnosis. These patients are also prone to other autoimmune disorders such as Graves' disease, Hashimoto's thyroiditis, Addison's disease, vitiligo, celiac sprue, autoimmune hepatitis, myasthenia gravis, and pernicious anemia.

Idiopathic diabetes

Some forms of type 1 diabetes do not have a known etiology. Some patients have persistent insulinopenia and are prone to ketoacidosis but have no evidence of autoimmunity. Although only a minority of patients with type

1 diabetes fall into this category, most of those with it are of African or Asian ancestry. Individuals with this form of diabetes suffer from episodic ketoacidosis and show varying degrees of insulin deficiency between episodes. This form of diabetes is strongly hereditary, lacks immunological evidence of β-cell autoimmunity, and is unrelated to HLA. The absolute requirement for insulin replacement therapy in affected patients may come and go.

Type 2 diabetes (ranging from predominantly insulin resistance with relative insulin deficiency to predominantly impaired insulin secretion with insulin resistance)

This form of diabetes, which accounts for approximately 90-95% of diabetes patients, previously referred to as non-insulin-dependent diabetes, type 2 diabetes, or adult-onset diabetes, involves individuals who have insulin resistance and usually have a relative (rather than absolute) deficiency of insulin. At least initially and often throughout life, these individuals do not need insulin treatment to survive. There are probably many different causes of this form of diabetes. Although the specific etiology is unknown, there is no autoimmune destruction of β-cells, and patients do not have any other causes of diabetes listed above or below.

Most patients with this form of diabetes are obese, and obesity itself causes some degree of insulin resistance. Patients who are not obese according to traditional weight criteria may have an increased percentage of body fat distributed predominantly in the abdominal area. Ketoacidosis rarely occurs spontaneously in this type of diabetes; when observed, it usually occurs associated with stress from another illness, such as an infection. This form of diabetes often goes undiagnosed for many years because hyperglycemia develops gradually. In the earlier stages, it is often not severe enough for the patient to notice any of the classic symptoms of diabetes. Nevertheless, these patients are more likely to develop macrovascular and microvascular complications. While patients with this form of diabetes may have insulin levels that appear normal or elevated, higher blood glucose levels in these diabetic patients would be expected to lead to even higher insulin levels if their β-cell function were normal. Insulin secretion is thus defective in these patients and insufficient to compensate for insulin resistance. Insulin resistance can be improved by weight reduction and/or pharmacological treatment of hyperglycemia but rarely returns to normal. The risk of developing this form of diabetes increases with age, obesity, and lack of physical activity. It occurs more frequently in women with prior GDM and individuals with hypertension or dyslipidemia, and its frequency varies in different racial/ethnic subgroups. It is often associated with a strong genetic predisposition, more so than with the autoimmune form of type 1 diabetes. However, the genetics of this form of diabetes is complex and is not fully defined.

Other specific types of diabetes

Genetic defects of β-cells

Several forms of diabetes are associated with monogenetic defects in β-cell function. The onset of hyperglycemia at an early age (usually before 25) often characterizes these forms of diabetes. They are called maturity-onset diabetes of the young (MODY) and are characterized by impaired insulin secretion with minimal or no impairment of insulin action. They are inherited in an autosomal dominant manner. So far, abnormalities have been identified at six genetic loci on different chromosomes. The most common form is associated with mutations on chromosome 12 in a liver transcription factor called hepatocyte nuclear factor (HNF)-1α. The second form is associated with mutations in the glucokinase gene on chromosome 7p, resulting in a defective glucokinase molecule. Glucokinase converts glucose to glucose-6-phosphate, whose metabolism, on the other hand, stimulates insulin secretion by the β-cell. Thus, glucokinase serves as a "glucose sensor" for the β-cell. Due to defects in the glucokinase gene, elevated plasma glucose levels are necessary to induce normal levels of insulin secretion. Less common forms result from mutations in other transcription factors, including HNF-4α, HNF-1β, insulin promoter factor (IPF)-1, and NeuroD1.

It turned out that diabetes diagnosed in the first six months of life is not a typical type 1 autoimmune diabetes. This so-called neonatal diabetes can be temporary or permanent. The most common genetic defect causing transient disease is a defect in the ZAC/HYAMI imprint. At the same time, permanent neonatal diabetes is often a defect in the gene encoding the Kir6.2 subunit of the β-cell K ATP channel. The latter's diagnosis has implications because such children may be well treated with sulfonylureas.

Point mutations in mitochondrial DNA are associated with diabetes and deafness. The most common mutation occurs at position 3,243 in the leucine tRNA gene, resulting in an A-to-G transition. An identical lesion occurs in MELAS syndrome (mitochondrial myopathy, encephalopathy, lactic acidosis, and stroke-like syndrome); however, diabetes is not a part of this syndrome, suggesting different phenotypic manifestations of this genetic lesion.

Genetic abnormalities that lead to the inability to convert proinsulin to insulin have been identified in several families, and such traits are inherited in an autosomal dominant manner. The resulting glucose intolerance is mild. Similarly, the production of mutant insulin molecules with a resulting impaired binding to the receptor has also been identified in several families and is associated with an autosomal inheritance and only mildly impaired or even normal glucose metabolism.

Genetic defects in insulin action

There are unusual causes of diabetes that result from genetically determined abnormalities in insulin action. Metabolic abnormalities associated with insulin receptor mutations can range from hyperinsulinemia and mild hyperglycemia to severe diabetes. Some individuals with these mutations may have acanthosis nigricans. Females may be virilized and have enlarged, cystic ovaries. In the past, this syndrome was called insulin resistance type A. Leprechaunism, and Rabson-Mendenhall syndrome are two childhood syndromes that have mutations in the insulin receptor gene with subsequent changes in insulin receptor function and extreme insulin resistance. The former is associated with characteristic facial features and is usually fatal in childhood, while the latter is associated with tooth and nail abnormalities and pineal hyperplasia.

Changes in insulin receptor structure and function cannot be proven in patients with insulin-resistant lipoatrophic diabetes. Therefore, it is assumed that the lesion(s) must be located in the post-receptor signal transduction pathways.

Diseases of the exocrine pancreas

Any process that diffusely damages the pancreas can cause diabetes. Acquired processes include pancreatitis, trauma, infection, pancreatectomy, and pancreatic cancer. Except for those caused by cancer, damage to the pancreas must be extensive for diabetes to appear; adrenocarcinomas, which affect only a small part of the pancreas, are associated with diabetes. This implies a different mechanism than a simple decrease in β-cell mass. If cystic fibrosis and hemochromatosis are extensive enough, they will also damage β-cells and impair insulin secretion. Fibrocalculous pancreatopathy may be accompanied by abdominal pain radiating to the back and pancreatic calcifications identified by X-ray examination. Pancreatic fibrosis and calcium stones in the exocrine ducts were found during the autopsy.

Endocrinopathies

Several hormones (e.g., growth hormone, cortisol, glucagon, epinephrine) antagonize the action of insulin. Excess of these hormones (e.g., acromegaly, Cushing's syndrome, glucagonoma, pheochromocytoma, in that order) can cause diabetes. This generally occurs in individuals with preexisting defects in insulin secretion, and hyperglycemia typically resolves when the excessive hormone levels are fixed.

Somatostatinomas and aldosteronoma-induced hypokalemia can cause diabetes, at least in part, by inhibiting insulin secretion. Hyperglycemia generally resolves after the successful removal of the tumor.

Diabetes caused by drugs or chemicals

Many medications can impair insulin secretion. These drugs may not cause diabetes alone but may induce diabetes in individuals with insulin resistance. In such cases, classification is unclear because the sequence or relative importance of β-cell dysfunction and insulin resistance is unknown. Certain toxins, such as Vacor (rat poison) and intravenous pentamidine, can permanently destroy pancreatic β-cells. Fortunately, such drug interactions are rare. Many drugs and hormones can also impair the effect of insulin. Examples include nicotinic acid and glucocorticoids. Patients receiving α-interferon have been reported to develop diabetes associated with anti-islet cell antibodies and, in some cases, severe insulin deficiency. The list shown in Table 2.1 is not complex but reflects the more commonly recognized drug, hormone, or toxin-induced forms of diabetes.

Infections

Some viruses are associated with β-cell destruction. Diabetes occurs in patients with congenital rubella, although most have HLA and immune markers characteristic of type 1 diabetes. In addition, coxsackie B virus, cytomegalovirus, adenovirus, and mumps have been implicated in causing some cases of the disease.

Less common forms of immune-related diabetes

There are two known conditions in this category, and there is a probability of even more occurring. Stiff-person syndrome is an autoimmune disease of the central nervous system characterized by stiffness of the axial muscles with

Table 2.1 Etiologic classification of diabetes mellitus (Source: Department of Vascular Surgery VUSCH)

I. Type 1 diabetes (β-cell destruction, usually leading to absolute insulin deficiency)	A, Immune-mediated
	B, Idiopathic
II. Type 2 diabetes (may range from predominantly insulin resistance with relative insulin deficiency to a predominantly secretory defect with insulin resistance)	
III. Other specific types	A, Genetic defects of β-cell function
	1. MODY 3 (Chromosome 12, HNF-1α) 2. MODY 1 (Chromosome 20, HNF-4α) 3. MODY 2 (Chromosome 7, glucokinase) 4. Other very rare forms of MODY (e.g., MODY 4: Chromosome 13, insulin promoter factor-1; MODY 6: Chromosome 2, *NeuroD1*; MODY 7: Chromosome 9, carboxyl ester lipase) 5. Transient neonatal diabetes (most commonly ZAC/HYAMI imprinting defect on 6q24) 6. Permanent neonatal diabetes (most commonly KCNJ11 gene encoding Kir6.2 subunit of β-cell K_{ATP} channel) 7. Mitochondrial DNA 8. Others
	B, Genetic defects in insulin action
	1. Type A insulin resistance 2. Leprechaunism 3. Rabson-Mendenhall syndrome 4. Lipoatrophic diabetes 5. Others
	C, Diseases of the exocrine pancreas
	1. Pancreatitis 2. Trauma/pancreatectomy 3. Neoplasia 4. Cystic fibrosis 5. Hemochromatosis 6. Fibrocalculous pancreatopathy 7. Others
	D, Endocrinopathies

(*Continued*)

Table 2.1 (Continued)

	1. Acromegaly 2. Cushing's syndrome 3. Glucagonoma 4. Pheochromocytoma 5. Hyperthyroidism 6. Somatostatinoma 7. Aldosteronoma 8. Others
	E, Drug or chemical induced
	1. Vacor 2. Pentamidine 3. Nicotinic acid 4. Glucocorticoids 5. Thyroid hormone 6. Diazoxide 7. β-Adrenergic agonists 8. Thiazides 9. Dilantin 10. γ-Interferon 11. Others
	F, Infections
	1. Congenital rubella 2. Cytomegalovirus 3. Others
	G, Uncommon forms of immune-mediated diabetes
	1. "Stiff-man" syndrome 2. Anti-insulin receptor antibodies 3. Others
	H, Other genetic syndromes sometimes associated with diabetes
	1. Down syndrome 2. Klinefelter syndrome 3. Turner syndrome 4. Wolfram syndrome 5. Friedreich ataxia 6. Huntington chorea 7. Laurence-Moon-Biedl syndrome 8. Myotonic dystrophy 9. Porphyria 10. Prader-Willi syndrome 11. Others
IV, Gestational diabetes mellitus	

painful spasms. Patients usually have high titers of GAD autoantibodies, and approximately one-third develop diabetes.

Anti-insulin receptor antibodies can cause diabetes by binding to the insulin receptor, thereby blocking insulin binding to its receptor in target tissues. However, in some cases, these antibodies can act as insulin agonists after binding to the receptor and can thus cause hypoglycemia. Antibodies against the insulin receptor are occasionally found in patients with systemic lupus erythematosus and other autoimmune diseases. As in different conditions of extreme insulin resistance, patients with insulin receptor antibodies often have acanthosis nigricans. In the past, this syndrome was called type B insulin resistance.

Other genetic syndromes that are sometimes associated with diabetes

An increased incidence of diabetes accompanies many genetic syndromes. These include the chromosomal abnormalities of Down syndrome, Klinefelter syndrome, and Turner syndrome. Wolfram syndrome is an autosomal recessive disorder characterized by insulin-deficient diabetes and the absence of β-cells at autopsy. Other manifestations include diabetes insipidus, hypogonadism, optic atrophy, and nerve-related hearing loss.

Gestational diabetes mellitus - GDM

For many years, GDM was defined as any glucose intolerance with onset or first recognition during pregnancy. Although most cases resolve by delivery, the definition was applied regardless of whether or not the condition persisted after pregnancy. It did not exclude the possibility that unrecognized glucose intolerance may have preceded or started concurrently with pregnancy. This definition has facilitated a unified strategy for detecting and classifying GDM, but its limitations have been known for many years. As the ongoing epidemic of obesity and diabetes has led to more type 2 diabetes in women of reproductive age, the number of pregnant women with undiagnosed type 2 diabetes has increased.

After deliberations in 2008–2009, the International Association of Diabetes and Pregnancy Study Groups (IADPSG), an international consensus group with representatives from several obstetric and diabetes organizations, including the American Diabetes Association (ADA), recommended that according to standard criteria, women at high risk for diabetes at the first prenatal visit will receive a diagnosis of overt, non-gestational diabetes. Approximately 7%

of all pregnancies (ranging from 1 to 14%, depending on the population studied and the diagnostic tests used) are complicated by GDM, resulting in more than 200,000 cases yearly.

Categories of increased risk of diabetes

In 1997 and 2003, the Expert Committee on the Diagnosis and Classification of Diabetes Mellitus recognized a transitional group of individuals whose glucose levels did not meet the criteria for diabetes but were higher than levels considered normal. These people were defined as having impaired fasting glycemia (IFG) [fasting plasma glucose (FPG) 100 mg/dL (5.6 mmol/L) to 125 mg/dL (6.9 mmol/L)] or impaired glucose tolerance (IGT) [2-hour oral glucose tolerance test (OGTT) values 140 mg/dL (7.8 mmol/L) to 199 mg/dL (11.0 mmol/L)].

Individuals with IFG and/or IGT were referred to as having prediabetes, indicating a relatively high risk of developing diabetes in the future. IFG and IGT should not be considered as separate clinical entities but rather as risk factors for diabetes and cardiovascular disease. They can be observed as intermediate stages in any of the disease processes. IFG and IGT are associated with obesity (especially abdominal or visceral obesity), dyslipidemia with high triglycerides and/or low HDL cholesterol, and hypertension. A structured lifestyle intervention aimed at increasing physical activity and causing a 5–10% loss of body weight and some pharmacological agents have been able to prevent or delay the development of diabetes in people with IGT; the potential impact of such interventions on reducing mortality or the incidence of cardiovascular disease has not yet been demonstrated. It should be noted that the 2003 ADA Expert Committee Report lowered the lower FPG threshold for defining IFG from 110 mg/dL (6.1 mmol/L) to 100 mg/dL (5.6 mmol/L), in part to ensure that the prevalence of IFG is similar to IGT.

Diagnostic criteria for diabetes mellitus

For decades, the diagnosis of diabetes was based on glucose criteria, either FPG or 75-g oGTT. In 1997, the first expert committee on the diagnosis and classification of diabetes mellitus revised the diagnostic criteria, using the observed association between FPG levels and the presence of retinopathy as a critical factor in identifying the threshold glucose level. The committee reviewed data from three cross-sectional epidemiologic studies that assessed retinopathy by fundus photography or direct ophthalmoscopy and measured glycemia as FPG, 2-h PG, and A1C. These studies demonstrated glycemic levels below which there was a negligible prevalence of retinopathy and above which the prevalence of retinopathy increased apparently linearly. The deciles of the three measures at which retinopathy began to grow were the same for each measure within each population. Furthermore, the glycemic values above which retinopathy increased were similar between patient populations. These analyses confirmed a long-term diagnostic 2-hour PG value ≥200 mg/dl (11.1 mmol/l). However, the older diagnostic FPG cutoff value of 140 mg/dL (7.8 mmol/L) has been reported to identify fewer individuals with diabetes than the 2-hour PG cutoff value. The FPG diagnostic threshold was lowered to ≥126 mg/dL (7.0 mmol/L). Eight mmol/L was found to identify far fewer individuals with diabetes than the 2-hour PG cutoff value.

A1C is a widely used marker of chronic glycemia that reflects average blood glucose levels over a 2- to 3-month period. The test plays a critical role in managing the patient with diabetes because it correlates well with microvascular and, to a lesser extent, with macrovascular complications and is widely used as a standard biomarker for the adequacy of glycemic management. Previous expert panels have not recommended using A1C to diagnose diabetes, partly because of insufficient test standardization. However, A1C tests are now highly standardized, so their results can be temporarily uniformly applied across populations. In the recent report, the International Expert Committee, after an extensive review of established and emerging epidemiologic evidence, recommended using the A1C test to diagnose diabetes with a threshold ≥ 6.5%, and the ADA affirms this decision. An A1C diagnostic threshold of 6.5% is associated with an inflection point in retinopathy prevalence and diagnostic thresholds for FPG and 2-h PG. The diagnostic test should be performed using a method certified by the National Glycohemoglobin Standardization Program (NGSP) and standardized or linked to the Diabetes Control and Complications Trial reference test. Point-of-care A1C tests are not currently accurate enough for diagnostic purposes.

There is a natural logic to using a more chronic-phase versus an acute-phase marker of dysglycemia, especially since A1C is already well-known to clinicians as a marker of glycemic control. In addition, A1C has several advantages over FPG, including greater convenience, as fasting is not required, evidence suggesting greater preanalytical stability, and fewer day-to-day disruptions during periods of stress and illness. However, these advantages must be balanced by higher costs, limited availability of A1C testing in some areas of the developing world, and the imperfect correlation between A1C and mean glucose levels in specific individuals. In addition, A1C can be misleading in patients with certain anemia and hemoglobinopathies, which may also have a unique ethnic or geographic distribution. In conditions with abnormal red blood cell turnover, such as hemolytic and iron deficiency anemias, only glucose criteria must be used to diagnose diabetes.

The established glucose criteria for the diagnosis of diabetes remain valid. These include FPG and 2-h PG. In addition, patients with severe hyperglycemia, such as those with severe classic hyperglycemic symptoms or hyperglycemic crisis, may continue to be diagnosed when a plasma glucose ≥ 200 mg/dL (11.1 mmol/L) is incidentally (or coincidentally) detected. In such cases, the healthcare professional would likely measure the A1C as a part of the initial assessment of diabetes severity, and it would (in most cases) be above the diagnostic cutoff value for diabetes. However, in rapidly developing diabetes, such as the development of type 1 diabetes in some children, A1C may not be significantly elevated at all.

On the other hand, if two different tests are available for an individual and the results are discordant, the test whose result is above the diagnostic limit should be repeated. The diagnosis should be made based on the confirmed test. This means that if a patient meets the criterion for diabetes with A1C (two results ≥6.5%) but does not meet the FPG criterion (<126 mg/dL or 7.0 mmol/L), or vice versa, that person should be considered diabetic. It is true that in most cases, the "non-diabetic" test is likely to be in the range very close to the threshold that defines diabetes.

The decision as to which test to use to assess a particular patient for diabetes should be at the healthcare professional's discretion, considering the availability and practicality of testing the individual patient or group of patients. Probably more important than the choice of diagnostic test used is that diabetes testing is done when indicated. There is discouraging evidence suggesting that many at-risk patients still do not receive adequate testing and counseling for this increasingly occurring disease or its often associated cardiovascular risk factors.

Screening and diagnosis of GDM

These new criteria will significantly increase the prevalence of GDM, primarily because only one abnormal value is sufficient to establish the diagnosis, not two of them. The ADA recognizes the anticipated significant increase in the incidence of GDM to be diagnosed under these criteria. It is sensitive to concerns about the "medicalization" of pregnancies previously categorized as normal. These changes to diagnostic criteria come in the context of alarming global increases in obesity and diabetes rates to optimize pregnancy outcomes for women and their babies.

After clinical studies in the 1970s, the next logical step was to use HbA 1c to evaluate whether improving glycemic control in diabetic patients can reduce long-term small-vessel (microvascular) and large-vessel (macrovascular) complications of diabetes. Two pivotal studies, the Diabetes Control and Complications Trial (DCCT) and the United Kingdom Prospective Diabetes Study (UKPDS), set out to determine the impact on microvascular complications in patients with type 1 (insulin-dependent) and type 2 (non-insulin-dependent) diabetes or it was hoped that these studies could also clarify whether macrovascular complications could be avoided in this way.

Traditionally, HbA 1c has been thought to represent average blood glucose over the past six to eight weeks. In fact, hemoglobin glycation occurs during the entire 120-day life of red blood cells, but during these 120 days, recent glycemia has the most significant impact on the HbA 1c value. Indeed, theoretical models and clinical studies suggest that in a patient with stable control, 50% of HbA 1c is formed in the month before sampling, 25% is formed in the month before that, and the remaining 25% is formed in months two to four. The advantage that HbA 1c can provide an assessment of average plasma glucose can also be seen as a disadvantage, as it does not indicate the stability of glycemic control. Theoretically, one patient with wildly fluctuating glucose concentrations could have the same HbA1c value as a patient whose glucose changes little during the day.

Some authors support the idea that HbA 1c testing is a more physiological assessment of glucose intolerance than the artificial states of the oGTT and therefore believe that it should be the preferred diagnostic test. Some studies have shown that HbA 1c is as good a predictor of microvascular disease as fasting or two-hour post-OGTT glucose values, although not all studies have reached this conclusion. One group took a more pragmatic approach to diagnosis, stating that subjects with an HbA1c of less than 7.0% were unlikely to require pharmacological treatment of their condition and, therefore, need not be classified as diabetic. However, the meta-analysis that derived the value of 7% did not conclusively account for the differences in HbA 1c methods between individual studies.

Microvascular complications

Microvascular (small blood vessel) complications of diabetes include retinopathy, nephropathy, and, most likely, neuropathy. Diabetic patients who develop these conditions constitute a large proportion of all subjects who develop blindness, renal failure, and/or require limb amputation. To investigate the effect that improving glycemic control may have on the development and progression of these complications, the DCCT study enrolled 1,441 young patients (mean age 27 years) with type 1 diabetes, half of whom were assigned to "conventional" treatment in the USA at the time (one or two insulin injections per day and daily urine/blood glucose monitoring), while the other half were assigned to "intensive" treatment (three or more insulin injections/day or an external pump and multiple daily blood glucose monitoring), where the goal was to achieve as close to normal blood glucose concentrations as possible. Hemoglobin A measurement 1C was the cornerstone of glycemic assessment in these patients. Compared to the non-diabetic reference range of 4.05% to 6.05%, the intensively treated group achieved a median HbA 1c of 7%, while the conventionally treated group achieved 9% during the study period. After a mean follow-up period of 6.5 years, the risk of retinopathy in the intensively treated group was reduced by 76%, the risk of proteinuria was decreased by 54%, and the risk of clinical neuropathy was reduced by 60%. The benefits extended to slowing the progression of retinopathy in patients who already had a mild form of eye disease at study entry.

Subsequent detailed analysis showed that the measurement of HbA 1c could be used to stratify the risk of developing microvascular complications in the patient, as the incidence of these complications increased exponentially with increasing HbA 1c values. This applied to all values of abnormal HbA 1c and not only 7% and 9%. Further examination also showed an apparent lack of a "glycemic threshold" - the lack of regular blood sugar – below which no small vessel complications occurred. Nevertheless, as with all exponential relationships, there was a law of diminishing returns, with the absolute benefit of lowering HbA 1c diminished as the initial value decreased. For example, the total reduction in risk of retinopathy in a patient whose HbA 1c drops from 7% to 5.2% is the same as that of another patient who declines from 10% to 9.7%. Striving for reasonable glycemic control by aiming for the lowest possible HbA 1c value is also not without risk. This study's rate of severe hypoglycemia increased exponentially with decreasing HbA 1c concentration. For many patients with diabetes, the fear of an acute complication such as hypoglycemia is greater than the possible increased risk of long-term small vessel complications due to chronically high HbA 1c values.

After the DCCT trial was reported in 1993, it was hoped, but not expected, that the results from this type 1 diabetes trial would equally apply to patients with type 2 disease, who represent most of the diabetic population. It took the publication of the UKPDS in 1998 to confirm that HbA 1c can also indicate the risk of small vessel complications in this group of patients. This study included 3,867 elderly patients (mean age 54 years) who were assigned either intensive treatment to achieve a fasting plasma glucose level of 6 mmol/L or conventional treatment to remain free of symptoms of hyperglycemia and/or to maintain fasting glucose below 15 mmol/liter. Again, HbA1c was measured using the same test used in the DCCT as the basis for treatment evaluation.

Differences between the groups were not so impressive this time as in DCTT (HbA 1c 7.0% vs. 7.9% in 10 years), but there was still a 25% decrease in microvascular endpoints risk in accordance with DCCT predictions.

The UKPDS may also have unintentionally indicated whether the stability of glycemic control and not just mean plasma glucose level influences the risk of small vessel disease because some patients were treated with insulin while others received sulfonylurea drugs. Because insulin-treated patients tend to have more significant glucose oscillations than non-insulin-treated patients, it was expected that the risk of complications at any HbA 1c value would be different between the two groups. There seemed to be no such differences.

These two recent studies have demonstrated the utility of measuring HbA 1c in predicting the risk of microvascular complications. As a result, they have led to a widely spread recommendation for its increased use. However, it should be emphasized that hyperglycemia, as measured by HbA 1c, is not the only contributor to this risk, as other factors may also have a significant influence. In the UKPDS – for example, a reduction in blood pressure from 154/87 to 144/82 was associated with a 37% decrease in microvascular endpoints. There was also a clustering of microvascular diseases in families participating in the DCCT, suggesting an additional genetic influence on the development and progression of complications.

Macrovascular damage

Although diabetic microvascular complications account for a large proportion of the excess morbidity and mortality associated with diabetes, the major cause remains the consequences of large vessel (macrovascular) disease. Diabetes is associated with a two- to three-fold increased risk of coronary heart disease in men and a four- to five-fold increased risk in premenopausal women. The DCCT and UKPDS studies did not primarily aim to determine whether there was a relationship between HbA 1c and heart disease. Still, a subgroup analysis was nevertheless performed to examine this question. In the DCCT, the rate of cardiovascular events was low because of the age of the patients enrolled. However, there was still an excess of macrovascular events in the conventional group compared with the intensive group (40 vs. 23), although this did not reach significance ($p = 0.08$). In the UKPDS, the incident rate was higher. Still, the separation of HbA 1c between the two groups was lower, and the findings were again statistically suggestive but not conclusive ($p = 0.052$ for myocardial infarction). However, a recent analysis showed that when the full range of HbA 1c concentrations in UKPDS patients is considered, a highly significant relationship exists between HbA 1c and the risk of coronary heart disease in these patients. Thus, HbA 1c indicates macrovascular risk (in addition to hypertension, smoking, etc.) in patients with diabetes and may, to some extent, indicate an excess risk of coronary events associated with the disease.

Metabolic disorders in diabetes mellitus affect various organ systems and can lead to end-organ failure. Although most musculoskeletal complications (MSC) of diabetes mellitus are usually not life-threatening, they often cause significant morbidity. While some MSCs have a proven association with diabetes mellitus, others are loosely associated due to their frequent coexistence, as are rheumatological complications. While many of these conditions are well known, some are overlooked in routine clinical practice. This text highlights key imaging features of less frequent MSCs and diabetes mellitus associations.

Diabetic complications and MSC associations will be discussed in the following categories:

1. Muscular: diabetic muscle ischemia; infectious and inflammatory myositis, denervation myositis.
2. Rheumatological associations: adhesive capsulitis (frozen shoulder), limited joint mobility syndrome (diabetic cheiropathy), Dupuytren's contracture, trigger finger, reflex sympathetic dystrophy syndrome, carpal tunnel syndrome.
3. Leg complications: necrobiosis lipoidica diabeticorum, Charcot joint, osteomyelitis, septic arthritis.
4. Spinal: diabetic neuropathic osteoarthropathy, diffuse idiopathic skeletal hyperostosis (DISH), dialysis-related spondyloarthropathy (amyloidosis).
5. Skin and soft tissues: cellulitis, necrotizing fasciitis, gas gangrene.

Diabetes-related muscle disorders

Diabetic myopathy may involve some or all of the following – muscle inflammation, fibrosis, atrophy, ischemia, infarction, hemorrhage, and necrosis. Using this general terminology can be confusing and should be avoided. Infectious myositis is a well-known pathology involving the muscles of people with diabetes. Skeletal muscle is usually not susceptible to infarction because of its rich collateral blood supply. Inflammatory myositis and denervation myositis can also occur in diabetics.

Diabetic muscle ischemia (DMI)

Also known as diabetic muscle infarction or diabetic myonecrosis, it is one of the rare complications in poorly controlled long-term diabetics and is usually a self-limiting condition. It is essential to recognize diabetic muscle ischemia because it is generally underreported and underappreciated. Clinical manifestations include the sudden onset of severe pain in the thigh or calf. Non-traumatic swelling of the affected limb is noted, which may persist for months. The traditional findings of fever and elevated white blood cell count are usually absent. Multiple muscles are often involved. The quadriceps, hip adductors, and hamstrings are the most commonly affected muscles. Bilateral involvement was reported in 8.4% of cases and is usually seen in poorly controlled long-standing diabetes mellitus. Failure of end-organs is quite common due to microvascular disease in this subset of patients. Imaging methods (CT, ultrasound, and X-rays) are non-specific. MR shows characteristic edematous muscle, although edema is a nonspecific finding. Hyperintensity on unenhanced T1-weighted images may represent hemorrhagic infarction. When a contrast substance is administered, the muscle may show central areas of hypoenhancement or non-enhancement, representing areas of infarction. Another pattern is heterogeneous areas with linear enhancing bands passing through a non-enhancing central zone enclosed in large regions of enlarging muscle. MRI also helps in identifying the site for biopsy if needed. Excisional biopsy is not recommended due to the increased risk of bleeding. Other causes of muscle edema, such as post-traumatic muscle contusions, subacute denervation, radiotherapy, compartment syndrome, polymyositis, infectious myositis, deep vein thrombosis, and rhabdomyolysis, should be ruled out. Although diabetic myonecrosis has a good short-term local prognosis, it overall indicates a poor long-term prognosis due to chronic vascular compromise.

Infectious myositis

Diabetes mellitus increases susceptibility to infection. Pyomyositis refers to infection of skeletal muscle, usually through hematogenous spread. However, blood cultures are positive at the time of presentation in only 5–35% of cases, and the most common cause is Staphylococcus aureus. Ultrasound helps in the detection of abscesses and edema. CT shows increased muscle volume and decreased attenuation due to edema. Intramuscular abscesses are perceived as a central zone of low attenuation with medium to high attenuation of the peripheral pseudocapsule and edge enhancement in post-contrast images. Necrotic tumor and intramuscular hematoma are in the differential diagnosis.

Denervation myositis

Subacute denervation causes uniform muscle edema, usually 2–4 weeks after the denervation event. Edema is said to be caused by the movement of intracellular water into the extracellular compartment. Muscle atrophy and fatty infiltration are signs of chronic denervation.

Rheumatological manifestations

Many rheumatological manifestations associated with diabetes mellitus affect the quality of life but are often overlooked in routine clinical practice. Sustained high blood sugar concentration leads to increased advanced glycosylation of end products, which are involved in promoting increased collagen cross-linking, which in turn reduces collagen flexibility, leading to increased stiffness of collagen and the structures built on the collagen framework, such as tendons, making them more vulnerable to contractures. In addition, there is an accumulation of collagen in the skin and periarticular connective tissue.

"Frozen shoulder" (adhesive capsulitis)

The prevalence of frozen shoulder in diabetic patients is 11–30%, with an estimated prevalence of 2–10% in nondiabetics. The joint capsule is thickened and closely approximates the head of the humerus, resulting in a loss of joint space. Three visible phases are recognized: painful, adhesive, and disappearing. In conventional shoulder arthrography, pain after injection of a small volume of contrast substance (less than 10 ml) is considered diagnostic. Thickening of the joint capsule in the axillary recess is associated with adhesive capsulitis. Other significant findings are synovitis in the anterosuperior glenohumeral joint and obliteration of the fatty triangle inferior to the coracoid process. MR shows no characteristic features, but for diagnosis, it is preferred when the thickness of the capsule and synovial lining in the axillary recess is greater than 3 mm, measured in a coronal fat-free, saturated sequence. A study by Song et al. found that soft tissue enlargement in the rotator interval and soft tissue and capsule thickening and enlargement in the axillary recess were suggestive of adhesive capsulitis on MRI.

Diabetic cheiroarthropathy (stiff hand syndrome)

Clinical features include limited joint mobility, thickened, stiff, waxy skin of the dorsal hand, and flexion contractures of the fingers. The thickening of the flexor tendon sheaths and subcutaneous tissue can be seen on ultrasound. Thickening and enlargement of the flexor tendon sheaths can be seen on MRI.

Dupuytren's contracture

Findings include focal thickening and shortening of the superficial palmar aponeurosis, leading to tethering and flexion contractures of the hands. Halesha et al. reported a 20 to 63% prevalence of Dupuytren's contracture in diabetic patients, a significant increase compared to the prevalence observed in the general population (13%). In diabetic patients, the middle and ring fingers are affected more often. Diagnostic imaging findings include nodularity with tethering involving the palmar aspect of the hand and finger, pre-tendon band, and flexion digital contracture. Ultrasound of the palmar fascia in Dupuytren's contracture may demonstrate knots and cords in the distal palmar crease. It usually affects the third and fourth fingers. The superficial palmar aponeurosis is a thin flat, superficial band of soft tissue located deep in the skin. The critical finding appears to be hypoechoic bands adjacent to the edges of the flexor tendons and the deep surface of the dermis. Initially, the nodules are hypoechoic and usually hypervascular. Over time, the nodules become more echogenic and lose vascularity. Arterial covering with fibrous or scar tissue can also be visualized with ultrasound. On MR, subcutaneous nodules are usually identified as cords running parallel and superficial to the flexor tendons in the distal palmar crease.

Reflex sympathetic dystrophy (RSD)

Reflex sympathetic dystrophy (RSD) is also known as complex regional pain syndrome (CRPS). Uncontrolled hyperglycemia can affect the occurrence of CRPS. In the study by Choi et al., as HbA1c values increased, the prevalence of CRPS increased, highlighting the association with diabetes mellitus in these

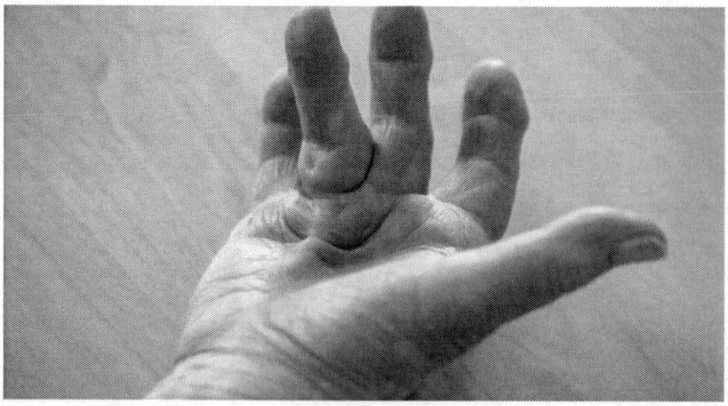

Figure 2.1 Dupuytren's contracture (Source: Department of Vascular Surgery VUSCH).

patient groups. The main clinical symptoms are pain, vasomotor symptoms, swelling, hyperhidrosis, hair changes, impaired mobility, tremor, and muscle spasms in the affected area. This usually improves after sympathetic denervation. Three stages are described.

Stage 1 (acute): plain X-rays show patchy, irregular bone loss.
Stage 2 (dystrophic): plain X-rays show diffuse bone loss that appears as diffuse ground glass.
Stage 3 (atrophic): disuse atrophy changes overlay stage 3 changes

However, these stages are poorly defined clinically or radiologically and may not help guide treatment or provide prognostic information. MR demonstrates bone marrow edema in RSD, a non-specific finding. In the study by Marko et al., MR images in stage 1 RSD showed thickening of periarticular, subcutaneous tissues and skin with occasional muscle and fascial edema. Stages 2 and 3 showed no contrast enhancement. Muscle atrophy was observed in stage 3, which was considered a sign of irreversibility. MR is, therefore, helpful in stages 1 and 3. It is known that RSD happens to recur.

Carpal Tunnel Syndrome (CTS)

Carpal tunnel syndrome (CTS) is thought to result from compression of the median nerve in the wrist deep to the transverse carpal ligament. The prevalence of CTS in people with diabetes is reportedly 13–49%, significantly more than in non-diabetics (1.6–13%). Nerve conduction studies may be helpful. Imaging is often used to look for space-occupying lesions such as flexor tenosynovitis, ganglia, masses, and gouty tophi deposits in the carpal tunnel and evaluate residual scarring or fibrosis in postoperative cases. The characteristic diagnostic ultrasound findings of carpal tunnel syndrome are a swollen nerve in the distal skin crease, just proximal to the carpal tunnel, flattening of the nerve in the distal tunnel, and palmar buckling of the transverse carpal ligament. The diagnosis should be considered when the maximum cross-sectional area of the focally enlarged median nerve is bigger than 0.09 cm2 at the wrist (any level). Nerve enlargement is measured where the nerve appears maximally enlarged and often corresponds to the level of the pisiform bone.

It is known that there is a subjective assessment of reduced sliding of the median nerve in the transverse plane, deep to the flexor retinaculum, during the index finger flexion and extension. It was concluded by Klauser et al. that an increase in median nerve cross-sectional area of 2 mm2 between proximal (measured at the proximal pronator quadratus) and distal (measured just

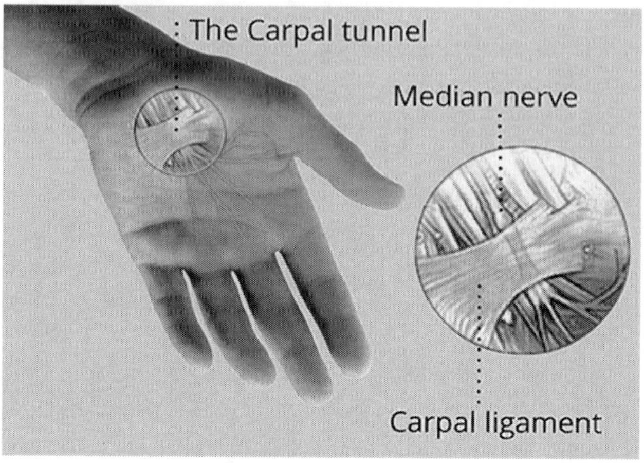

Figure 2.2 Schematic representation of carpal tunnel syndrome (source: Department of Vascular Surgery VUSCH).

proximal to the inlet of the flexor retinaculum) provides 99% sensitivity and 100% specificity for the carpal tunnel syndrome diagnosis.

Hyperintensity of the nerve is recorded on fat-suppressed T2 weighted images or short-tau inversion recovery (STIR). Postoperative examination mainly includes an assessment of the appearance of the nerve and its ability to slide freely under the retinaculum. Moreover, a retinaculum tear can be seen. Postoperative symptoms may be caused by inadequate retinaculum resection. Another complication and cause of the late return of symptoms is scar tissue formation.

Foot complications

The diabetic foot is prone to infection, ulceration, neuroarthropathy, and fractures. In these groups of patients, wound healing is a challenge. It is estimated that people with diabetes have a 15% lifetime risk of developing a foot ulcer. The ten-year cumulative incidence of lower extremity amputation is estimated to be 5 to 7% in diabetic foot. Imaging is essential in diagnosing infection/osteomyelitis/abscess, ulcer depth, joint/tendon exposure to the wound, ischemia, and gangrene.

Necrobiosis lipoidica diabeticorum

The incidence of Necrobiosis lipoidica diabeticorum ranges from 0.3 to 1.6% of diabetics per year. It is a soft tissue disorder caused by microangiopathy that often presents as confluent, painless red cutaneous papules that form granulomatous masses in the pretibial region and along the dorsum of the foot. They can later infiltrate the adjacent bone or disappear spontaneously. The diagnosis is established by clinical examination. However, high-frequency ultrasound would help us identify foci of inflammation in the middle and deep dermis and localize the presence of panniculitis with edema. Hypoechoic areas, which can be seen, often represent dermal inflammation, with increased blood flow on color Doppler, as studied by Gracia et al. in a patient with necrobiosis lipoidica but in a patient without diabetes.

Charcot's joints

Charcot's joints occur in up to 15% of people with diabetes. Peripheral neuropathy results in a lack of proprioception and pain perception. Damage to the joint and ligaments can be caused by normal weight-bearing activities, further increasing the malignancy and leading to abnormal mobility and progressive breakdown. It is assumed that progressive changes from hypervascularization to non-vascularity contribute to trophic changes. Weight-bearing joints (tarsometatarsal and intertarsal joints) are mainly affected. Other joints, such as the spine, knees, and upper limbs, are affected less often. The six Ds noted in Charcot's joint are increased bone Density, joint Distension, joint Disorganization, Debris (bone fragments), joint Destruction, and Dislocation. In chronic neuropathic osteoarthropathy, MR has a characteristically reduced signal intensity in the bone marrow, consistent with osteosclerosis on all sequences and cystic lesions in the bone marrow. The consequences may be hammer toes and collapse of the middle tarsus.

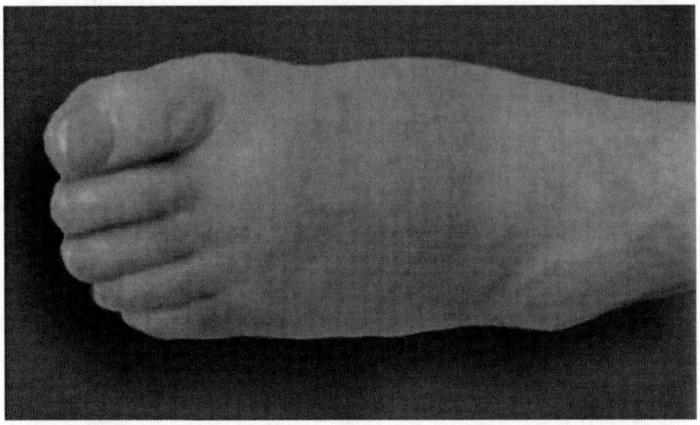

Figure 2.3 Formation of Charcot joints in diabetes mellitus (source: Department of Vascular Surgery VUSCH).

Recent rapidly progressive neuropathic osteoarthropathy is a close mimic of osteomyelitis. MRI shows low signal intensity on T1 in the bone marrow and high signal intensity on T2 weighted MR images. Recent fractures associated with a neuropathic joint can cause signal changes in the marrow and cortex. In this setting, soft tissue infection complicates the diagnosis when distinguishing osteomyelitis from acute neuropathic changes.

Osteomyelitis

Osteomyelitis occurs in up to 15% of people with diabetes. Osteomyelitis is an infection of the bone marrow, while infectious osteitis refers to an infection of the cortex, and infectious periostitis is an infection of the periosteum. Common imaging findings include soft tissue and bone marrow edema, periostitis, erosions, and osteopenia. Chronic osteomyelitis manifests itself as bone sclerosis, islands of dead bone (sequestration). X-rays are insensitive in the early stages and take weeks (7–15 days) to demonstrate cortical destruction and periostitis. MRI is the examination of choice (sensitivity 90% and specificity 83%) for detecting osteomyelitis of the foot and soft tissue infection. STIR is the most sensitive diagnostic imaging modality, while bone marrow hyperintensity on STIR corresponds to T1 hypointensity. STIR hyperintensity without significant T1 hypointensity may represent only edematous changes due to hyperemia related to soft tissue infection. Paul et al. emphasized that STIR, T2-weighted, and contrast-enhanced sequences should be interpreted with findings on T1-weighted images. They described a confluent pattern of decreased bone marrow signal on T1 images with medullary distribution correlated well with osteomyelitis. A limited inhomogeneous subcortical distribution of T1 signal changes of abnormal bone marrow signal on T1-weighted images does not suggest established osteomyelitis and likely represents reactive edema. Adjacent soft-tissue edema, ulcer, and abscess may occur. Differentiating viable tissue from non-enhancing non-viable tissue using a contrast study is essential, as this indicates the need for surgical debridement in addition to antibiotic therapy. Acute neuropathic arthropathy may be mimicked.

Multiple bone and joint involvement, periarticular and subchondral predilection, overlying intact skin, and absence of ulcers and sinus tracts favor the diagnosis of Charcot neuropathic joint rather than osteomyelitis. In chronic arthropathy, the differentiation is easy due to the lack of marrow edema; however, the disappearance of previously observed subchondral cysts or intra-articular bodies in patients with neuroarthropathy suggests a superimposed infection. Another feature noted by Ahmedi et al. is that the frequency of intra-articular loose bodies is lower in an infected neuropathic joint, probably due to the dissolution of these bodies after the onset of infection, or that their signal intensity may change to a fluid signal due to surrounding edema and become obscured.

Septic arthritis

The spread from the adjacent infected bone usually initiates joint infection. In the early stages, joint effusion, erosions, and periarticular osteopenia are common findings. Late changes include loss of joint space and destruction. Septic arthritis must be treated urgently because joint infection leads to rapid cartilage destruction with permanent joint loss. MR findings of septic arthritis include joint effusion, pericapsular edema, uniform cartilage destruction, bone erosion, marrow edema, synovitis, abscess, tendon/muscle infections, and pannus. MRI has a role, especially if sent for evaluation after a joint is drily tapped, to demonstrate loculated fluid, a pannus to support septic arthritis or to suggest another diagnosis.

Complications of the spine

Spinal neuroarthropathy

Diabetes mellitus is a significant contributor to chronic kidney disease (CKD). The estimated prevalence of CKD in adults with type 2 diabetes mellitus is 34.5–42.3%. In addition, diabetes is present in approximately 30-40% of all cases of end-stage renal disease in the USA. Spinal neuroarthropathy, also called Charcot's spine, is a condition resulting from progressive loss of pain perception and proprioception, leading to progressive aseptic destruction of the spine, including the disc, vertebral bodies, and facet joints. Tabes dorsalis, syringomyelia, traumatic brain, and spinal cord injury are other causes of Charcot's spine. Alexis et al. described two stages of Charcot spine development. First, nonspecific inflammatory-type changes occur in two adjacent endplates, mimicking disc degeneration ± inflammation. Vacuum phenomena may be present in disc and facet joints. In the second and last stage, the destruction of the end plates and the intervening disc with bone sclerosis and new bone formation is observed. Similar findings can also be noted with facet joints. Infection is a close mimic. Differentiating features of Charcot's spine include intradiscal vacuum phenomena with bone fragmentation, joint disorganization and dislocations, spondylolisthesis, and facet joint involvement. In Charcot's spine, the entire vertebral bodies show high-intensity signals on T 2-weighted sequences and postcontrast imaging, whereas, in infection, signal changes are usually limited to the endplates. Timely diagnosis and treatment at an earlier stage of inflammation are likely to lead to further destruction.

DISH (Forestier's disease) is commonly seen in diabetics, more often in type 2. The prevalence is 13–49% in diabetic patients and 1.6–13% in non-diabetics. It is thought that the prolonged high levels of insulin and insulin-like growth factors associated with diabetes mellitus may stimulate new bone growth. The aforementioned new bone formation occurs most often in the thoracolumbar vertebra, while the typical sign is the calcification of the spinal ligaments. In addition to the calcification of the anterior longitudinal ligament, posterior osteophytes and ossification of the posterior longitudinal ligament may also occur in the lower cervical spine. New bone formation characteristically appears as bony bridging between successive vertebral bodies. In the chest, it is more pronounced on the right side of the thoracic vertebra. In contrast, the deficiency on the left side is explained by inhibiting new bone formation due to a left-sided pulsating descending thoracic aorta. Criteria for the DISH diagnosis are the involvement of at least four adjacent vertebrae of the thoracic spine, usually with preserved intervertebral disc space, and the absence of inflammatory changes in the sacroiliac joints. Hyperostosis of the heel, elbow, and spine may be present. Extraspinal enthesopathy changes can be observed in the heel, patella, and pelvis. Treatment is usually conservative.

Amyloidosis and dialysis-associated spondyloarthropathy

The presence of diabetes mellitus among patients with end-stage renal disease is approximately 30–40%. Chronic kidney disease can lead to amyloidosis. Given this strong association, we have included a brief note on dialysis-associated amyloidosis and spondyloarthropathy in this review. Amyloid deposition occurs in 20% of patients who have undergone long-term hemodialysis. Amyloid deposition consists of β2-microglobulin. Amyloid can be deposited in the tendons and synovial sheaths around the carpal tunnel, leading to median nerve compression. Amyloid deposits can lead to radiolucent areas (dialysis cysts), usually present in the carpal bones, phalanges, humeral head, and around the hips, and may enlarge with continued dialysis. Bone imaging findings of amyloidosis include focal lytic lesions, endosteal indentation, osteopenia, and pathological fractures. Large soft tissue masses can cause the notching of adjacent bone. Long-term amyloidosis leads to extensive joint destruction.

Skin and soft tissue complications

Cellulitis

Skin and soft tissue complications are five times higher, and associated hospitalizations are four times higher in patients with diabetes than those without diabetes. Peripheral neuropathy can result in repeated unrecognized microtrauma with dry, cracked skin. This may initially manifest as callus formation, later as soft tissue injury, ulceration, and abscess formation. Peripheral vascular disease results in poor healing. Hyperglycemia leads to an altered immunological response to infection, and delays wound healing. Cellulitis is an infection of the skin and subcutaneous tissue usually caused by Gram-positive cocci. Ultrasound findings include subcutaneous edema, skin thickening, and hypervascularization with fluid surrounding the hyperechoic fat lobe and extending along the interlobular septa. Ultrasound also plays a crucial role in determining the patency of deep veins. Soft tissue enhancement in a postcontrast study is essential for differentiating cellulitis from simple edema caused by volume overload, congestive heart failure, or lymphatic obstruction.

Necrotizing fasciitis

Necrotizing fasciitis is a rapidly progressive infection centered around the deep fascia that progresses to tissue necrosis and systemic toxicity. Emergency surgery is necessary to save the limb. Nonspecific thickening of the fascia (>3 mm), edema, and enhancement of the fascia on contrast images are MR findings. The presence of gas in deep fascial planes, in the absence of penetrating trauma, ulceration, or recent surgery, is a strong indicator of necrotizing fasciitis under appropriate clinical circumstances and is better seen on CT or even X-rays. However, the presence of gas is not necessary for diagnosis as in the early stages; fascial and skin thickening are the only signs. In addition, it is not advisable to wait for an MRI, as this is a surgical emergency.

Gas gangrene

Gas gangrene is a rapidly progressive and life-threatening bacterial (often clostridial) infection and can lead to septicemia. The presence of gas bubbles in soft tissues is felt as crepitus on clinical examination and is diagnostic on plain films. Urgent surgical examination and administration of antibiotics are the treatment of choice. Cross-sectional imaging (CT, MRI) may delay surgical exploration and should only be included as a diagnostic tool with caution.

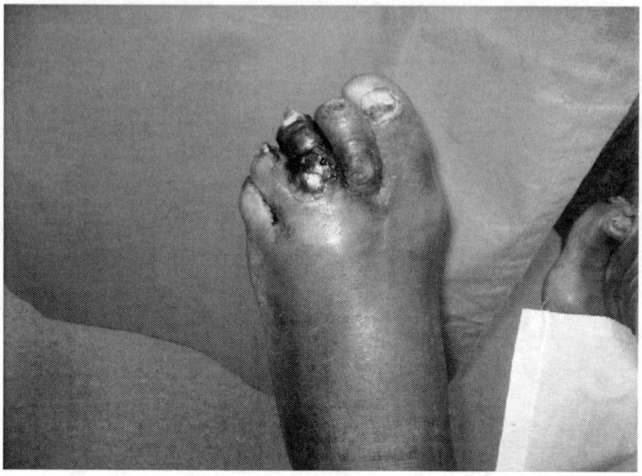

Figure 2.4 Gas gangrene of the left foot (Source: Department of Vascular Surgery VUSCH).

References

Ackermann RT, Cheng YJ, Williamson DF, Gregg EW. Identifying adults at high risk for diabetes and cardiovascular disease using hemoglobin A1c National Health and Nutrition Examination Survey 2005–2006. Am J Prev Med 2011;40:11–17

Brahee DD, Guebert GM, Virgin B. Dialysis-related spondyloarthropathy. J Manipulative Physiol Ther 2001; 24: 127–30. DOI: 10.1067/mmt.2001.112560.

Crowther CA, Hiller JE, Moss JR, McPhee AJ, Jeffries WS, Robinson JS. Vplyv liečby gestačného diabetes mellitus na výsledky tehotenstva . N Engl J Med 2005; 352 :2477–2486

Edelman D, Olsen MK, Dudley TK, Harris AC, Oddone EZ. Užitočnosť hemoglobínu A1c pri predpovedaní rizika cukrovky . J Gen Intern Med 2004; 19 :1175–1180

Geiss LS, Pan L, Cadwell B, Gregg EW, Benjamin SM, Engelgau MM. Changes in incidence of diabetes in U.S. adults, 1997–2003. Am J Prev Med 2006;30:371–377

Genuth S, Alberti KG, Bennett P, Buse J, DeFronzo R, Kahn R, Kitzmiller J, Knowler WC, Lebovitz H, Lernmark A, Nathan D, Palmer J, Rizza R, Saudek C, Shaw J, Steffes M, Stern M, Tuomilehto J, Zimmet P, Odborný výbor pre diagnostiku a klasifikáciu diabetu mellitus Správa o následnom diagnostikovaní diabetes mellitus . Diabetes Care 2003; 26 :3160–3167

Knowler WC, Barrett-Connor E, Fowler SE, Hamman RF, Lachin JM, Walker EA, Nathan DM, Diabetes Prevention Program Research Group Reduction in the incidence of type 2 diabetes with lifestyle intervention or metformin. N Engl J Med 2002;346:393–403

Landon MB, Spong CY, Thom E, Carpenter MW, Ramin SM, Casey B, Wapner RJ, Varner MW, Rouse DJ, Thorp JM, Jr., Sciscione A, Catalano P, Harper M, Saade G, Lain KY, Sorokin Y, Peaceman AM, Tolosa JE, Anderson GB. A multicenter, randomized trial of treatment for mild gestational diabetes. N Engl J Med 2009;361:1339–1348

Medzinárodný expertný výbor Správa Medzinárodného expertného výboru o úlohe testu A1C pri diagnostike diabetu . Diabetes Care 2009; 32 : 1327–1334

Metzger BE, Gabbe SG, Persson B, Buchanan TA, Catalano PA, Damm P, Dyer AR, Leiva A, Hod M, Kitzmiller JL, Lowe LP, McIntyre HD, Oats JJ, Omori Y, Schmidt MI. International Association of Diabetes and Pregnancy Study Group's recommendations on the diagnosis and classification of hyperglycemia in pregnancy. Diabetes Care 2010;33:676–682

Metzger BE, Lowe LP, Dyer AR, Trimble ER, Chaovarindr U, Coustan DR, Hadden DR, McCance DR, Hod M, McIntyre HD, Oats JJ, Persson B, Rogers MS, Sacks DA. Hyperglycemia and adverse pregnancy outcomes. N Engl J Med 2008;358:1991–2002

Murphey MD, Sartoris DJ, Quale JL, Pathria MN, Martin NL. Musculoskeletal manifestations of chronic renal insufficiency. Radiographics 1993; 13: 357–79. DOI: 10.1148/radiographics.13.2.8460225

Odborná komisia pre diagnostiku a klasifikáciu diabetes mellitus. Správa expertnej komisie pre diagnostiku a klasifikáciu diabetes mellitus . Diabetes Care 1997; 20 :1183–1197

Pradhan AD, Rifai N, Buring JE, Ridker PM. Hemoglobín A1c predpovedá diabetes, ale nie kardiovaskulárne ochorenie u nediabetických žien . Am J Med 2007; 120 :720–727

Sato KK, Hayashi T, Harita N, Yoneda T, Nakamura Y, Endo G, Kambe H. Kombinované meranie plazmatickej glukózy nalačno a A1C je účinné na predikciu diabetu 2. typu: Kansai Healthcare Study . Diabetes Care 2009; 32 : 644–646

Selvin E, Steffes MW, Zhu H, Matsushita K, Wagenknecht L, Pankow J, Coresh J, Brancati FL. Glycated hemoglobin, diabetes, and cardiovascular risk in nondiabetic adults. N Engl J Med 2010;362:800–811

Shimazaki T, Kadowaki T, Ohyama Y, Ohe K, Kubota K. Hemoglobin A1c (HbA1c) predicts future drug treatment for diabetes mellitus: a follow-up study using routine clinical data in a Japanese university hospital. Translational Research 2007;149:196–204

Suaya JA, Eisenberg DF, Fang C, Miller LG. Skin and soft tissue infections and associated complications among commercially insured patients aged 0-64 years with and without diabetes in the U.S. PLoS One 2013; 8: e60057. Doi: 10.1371/journal.pone.0060057

Theodorou DJ, Theodorou SJ, Resnick D. Imaging in dialysis spondyloarthropathy. Semin Dial 2002; 15: 290–6.

Turecki MB, Taljanovic MS, Stubbs AY, Graham AR, Holden DA, Hunter TB, et al. . Zobrazovanie infekcií muskuloskeletálnych mäkkých tkanív . Skeletal Radiol 2010; 39 : 957-971. doi: 10.1007/s00256-009-0780-0

Zhang X, Gregg EW, Williamson DF, Barker LE, Thomas W, Bullard KW, Imperatore G, Williams DE, Albright AL. A1C level and future risk of diabetes: a systematic review. Diabetes Care 2010;33:1665–1673.

Chapter 3

Etiology and Diagnostics of the Diabetic Foot

Jana Pobehová, MD*

Department of Vascular Surgery, East Slovak Institute of Cardiovascular Diseases, Košice, Slovakia

Abstract

Diabetic foot syndrome (DFS) combines chronic, long-term non-healing ulcerations on the skin, in any part of the leg, complicated by infection of soft tissues and phlegmon, which passes into deeper layers up to the bone, with the risk of developing osteomyelitis. The prevalence of DFS is up to 10%, and the incidence is up to 5.9%. Up to 15% of diabetes patients are exposed to the risk of leg ulceration. Up to ¼ of people with diabetes will develop a difficult-to-heal wound on the leg at least once in their life that requires long-term and expensive treatment, including hospitalizations and increased outpatient care. The prognosis of DFS may not always be bad if, after a proper diagnosis is followed by adequate treatment, the condition may not result in amputation. It is stated that a modern, multidisciplinary approach can reduce amputations by up to 43-86%. Treatment of diabetic ulcers represents a growing socio-economic burden.

Key Words: diabetic foot syndrome, ulceration, amputation, phlegmon, diabetic ulcer

Introduction

The WHO defines diabetic foot syndrome (DFS) as ulceration or tissue destruction distal to the ankle, including the ankle joint, associated with varying degrees of ischemia and neuropathy in diabetics. Infection is also often present.

---

* Corresponding Author's Email: jana.pastvova@post.cz

In: Diabetic Foot
Editor: Martina Zavacká
ISBN: 979-8-89113-019-7

It is characterized by chronic, long-term non-healing ulcerations on the skin in any part of the leg, complicated by infection of soft tissues and phlegm, which passes into the deeper layers of the bone, with the risk of osteomyelitis. Tissue necrosis can gradually develop – into gangrene, which leads to amputation of the affected part of the limb, depending on the blood supply.

The prevalence of DFS is up to 10%, and the incidence is up to 5.9%. Up to 15% of people with diabetes are exposed to the risk of leg ulcers during their lifetime. The most significant factor is diabetes mellitus, first diagnosed in 2.8% of patients hospitalized for leg problems and 15% admitted to the hospital for the need for limb amputation. Up to ¼ of people with diabetes develop a difficult-to-heal leg wound at least once in their lifetime, which requires long-term and expensive treatment, including hospitalization and increased outpatient care. In 2015, two million Americans underwent an amputation, most commonly due to diabetes and peripheral artery disease. Femoral amputation in the US reaches 40 per 100,000 patients with diabetes. Due in part to an aging population and an increase in the prevalence of people living with diabetes, it is believed that the number of Americans with amputations will have doubled by 2050. This growing population of US amputees has a higher prevalence of cardiovascular disease than the general adult population: up to 75% have coronary artery disease, 60–80% have hypertension, 15–25% have cerebrovascular disease, and 20–50% have congestive heart failure. By comparison, only about 37% of US adults have at least one type of cardiovascular disease. Cardiovascular disease remains the leading cause of death and health care expenditure in the USA, with direct and indirect costs reaching $316.1 billion in 2012-2013. Spending is expected to nearly triple by 2030, with much of this rising cost attributable to modifiable risk factors.

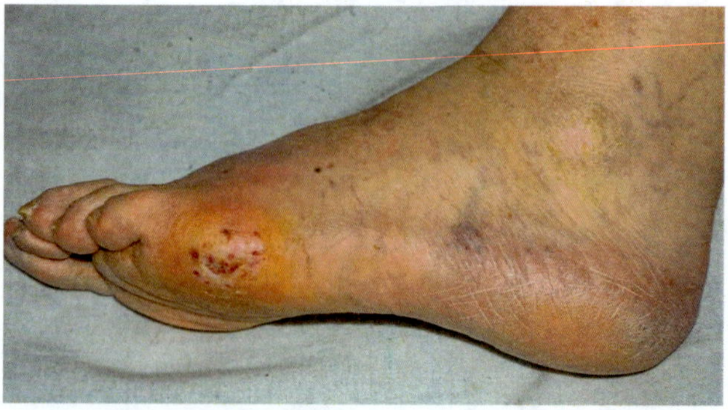

Figure 3.1 Diabetic foot (necrosis and ischemia of the foot - source: Department of Vascular Surgery VUSCH).

In developing countries, the numbers are much higher. The data are significantly underestimated in Slovakia as well. In 2011, Slovak diabetologists reported that 25.2% of patients had diabetic neuropathy, 2.31% had a diabetic leg with an ulcer, and 1.23% of people with diabetes underwent amputation. The prevalence of critical limb ischemia (CLI) is five times higher in people with diabetes than in non-diabetics. Some data indicate up to 20% incidence of CLI in people with diabetes with a dire prognosis. Diabetes causes up to 70% of all amputations, and almost 85% of all amputations are preceded by leg ulceration. However, it is the inevitable end of DFS. Early recognition of risk factors, preventive measures, and intensive treatment of complications significantly reduce the number of limb amputations in people with diabetes, considerably saving financial resources. Risk factors for diabetic foot syndrome include old age, high blood pressure, and smoking.

The main factors in developing DFS are diabetic neuropathy and ischemic disease of the lower limbs. In addition, infections and cheiroarthropathy (decreased joint mobility) are also involved. The final pathophysiological factors that lead to the formation of ulcerations are intravascular rheological and hemocoagulation changes, a decrease in tissue oxygenation, which induces biomechanical stress, or external traumatic stimuli are added. Other risk factors for ulceration are older age, male sex, European race, previous leg ulcers, and other microvascular complications of diabetes.

Diabetes mellitus is a growing public health problem with an increasing prevalence estimated at 3.6 million people in the UK, with an expected further increase to 5 million in the next ten years. A complication of the diabetic foot represents a significant health burden and the most common reason for hospitalization of diabetic patients. It is estimated that up to 2–3% of patients with diabetes mellitus have an active foot ulcer, with a lifetime risk of developing an ulcer of up to 25%.

About 50% of patients with diabetes mellitus will develop symptomatic peripheral neuropathy within 25 years of the onset of the disease. Patient age, disease duration, and quality of diabetes control are strong predictors, while etiology has no effect. Signs of autonomic neuropathy can be found in 20% of cases, again strongly correlated with age and disease duration, as well as with microangiopathy. Autonomic neuropathy accompanies peripheral neuropathy in 30% to 50% of cases. Distal symmetric sensorimotor neuropathy can be found in approximately 30% of hospitalized patients with diabetes mellitus (diabetes as a primary or secondary diagnosis) compared to 20% in the general diabetic population. Painful chronic polyneuropathy is reported by 13 to 26% of diabetes patients. It is estimated that more than two-thirds of non-traumatic lower extremity amputations are preceded by an ulcer (84%), a critical event that opens the window for early intervention.

Diabetes mellitus is commonly associated with a series of micro- and macrovascular changes manifesting as a broad spectrum of complications. Diabetic foot ulcers are the worst component of diabetes progression, with an estimated 15% of diabetic patients developing foot ulcers during their disease. Commonly identified risk factors predisposing to the development of leg ulcers include poor glycemic control, peripheral neuropathy, peripheral vascular disease, and immunosuppression.

In patients with ischemic disease of the lower limbs, there is a narrowing of the lumen of the arteries to the point of closure due to the deposition of acidic mucopolysaccharides in the artery wall. This is manifested by significant pain: initially when walking, then even at rest. Diabetic ulcers of ischemic origin are often excruciating and appear on the tips of the fingers, heel, or foot edge. If an artery is blocked, sharp pain will occur, which signals a lack of oxygen and nutrients in the tissues and muscles. The ischemic leg is also cold, purple, and without a palpable pulse on the periphery.

Up to 1/3 of people with diabetes are affected by either painful or painless neuropathy. If the limb loses sensitivity, deformities of the foot (in the case of a motor form of neuropathy) are associated, leading to its non-physiological load with the development of callosities (hyperkeratosis), subcutaneous bleeding, skin damage, and the formation of a defect. The absence of a feeling of pressure, pain, and discomfort for a person with diabetes helps the rapid development of DFS. Plantar overload, microtraumas, and joint mobility disorders

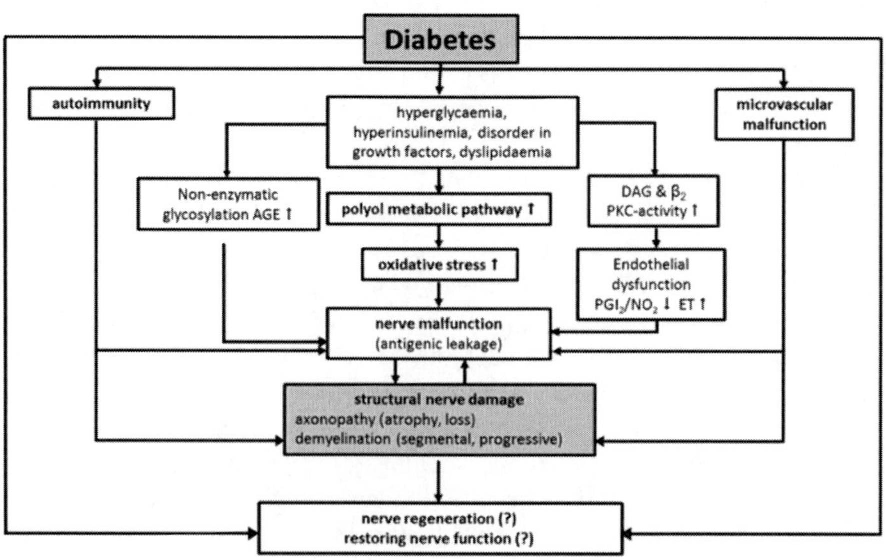

Figure 3.2 Diagram of the development of diabetes mellitus (source: Department of Vascular Surgery VUSCH).

lead to hyperkeratosis. Micro and macroangiopathy with varying degrees of leg tissue ischemia is just another part of the DFS puzzle. The development of autonomic neuropathy causes sweating disorders, dry skin, and edema. Boulton concluded that up to 85% of diabetic foot ulcers could be attributed to peripheral neuropathy that alters foot pressures.

The annual diabetic foot assessment recommended by the National Institute for Clinical Excellence requires that all people with diabetes have the following:

- Neurological testing of the foot: 10 g of monofilament at four sites on each foot and one of the following: vibration using a 128 Hz tuning fork, pinprick sensation, ankle reflexes, and vibration perception threshold;
- Foot shape: prominent metatarsal/claw toe heads, hallux valgus, muscle wasting, or Charcot deformity;
- Dermatological control: callus, erythema, and sweating;
- Vascular check: foot pulses, ankle-brachial index (if indicated), and Doppler waves.

Appropriate clinical examination of the diabetic foot can lead to the diagnosis of diabetic peripheral neuropathy. Clinical examination is also helpful in the classification and risk stratification of the disease for monitoring patients in outpatient clinics.

The biochemical basis of ulceration results from a combination of components that lead to tissue breakdown. Persistent hyperglycemic conditions lead to the complex formation of advanced glycation end products and cytokines, which induce oxidative stress on the nerve cell, leading to motor, autonomic, and sensory neuropathy. In addition, skin insensitivity resulting from autonomic changes that impair sweat gland function leads to further callus formation. Damaged sensorimotor neurons cause a reduced or altered sensation, further affecting walking mechanics.

Diagnosis of diabetes

The task of the diabetologist is to determine the correct diagnosis. It is determined based on anamnestic data, physical examination, and laboratory parameters. The most important is glycemia: physiological fasting level up to 7.0 mmol/l, at any time during the day, up to 11.1 mmol/l. It is necessary to determine them at least twice a row to exclude possible laboratory errors. Today it is valid that HbA1c should be up to 6.5%. An oGTT (oral glucose tolerance test) is performed in unclear cases. Three days before the test, the patient eats

Table 3.1 Pathogenesis of the development of the diabetic foot (adapted from Krahulec et al., 2003)

Neurogenic factors	Sensory denervation (loss of pain sensation)
	Motor denervation (muscle atrophy)
	Autonomic (sympathetic) denervation (anhidrosis, eczema)
	Osteoarthropathy - Charcot neuropathic osteoarthropathy
	Hyperkeratoses and callosities
Vascular factors	Macroangiopathy (narrowing of arteries, ischemia)
	Microcirculation (functional changes)
	Rheological and hemocoagulation changes in the vascular system
	Tissue hypoxia
Mechanical factors	Changed leg statics and bone deformities
	Abnormal pressure distribution, syndrome of limited joint mobility
	Excessive local load on the leg
	Trauma
Metabolic factors	Poor diabetes mellitus compensation
	Ketosis and ketoacidosis
	Duration of diabetes
	Non-enzymatic glycation of proteins
Factors causing infection	Injuries, bruises
	Trophic eczema
	Poor foot hygiene
	Fungal infection
Social factors	Low social level
	Poor availability of healthcare
	Non-compliance of the patient
Other factors	Older age of the patient
	Male
	Europoid race
	Previous leg ulcers
	Insufficient education

a regular diet with sufficient carbohydrate content. After a 10-hour fast, the patient drinks 75 g of glucose in 300 ml of water (flavored with lemon) within 3-5 minutes. Fasting blood glucose and the level after 120 minutes are decisive for the evaluation. Glycemia higher than 11.1 mmol/l after 120 minutes indicates a diagnosis of DM. If blood glucose is between 7.8-11.0 mmol/l, it is a glucose tolerance disorder, one of the pre-diabetes syndromes.

Management of diabetes

It is essential to determine the goal of treatment. Evaluate the patient's age, duration of diabetes, risk of DFS, and associated diseases. It should always be remembered that the better the metabolic compensation, the better the wound healing. If we have a patient with developed DFS, with developed chronic complications, according to the ACCORD study, aggressive treatment of hyperglycemia is not appropriate for these patients. According to the recommendations of the ADA (American Diabetes Association) and the EASD (European Association for the Study of Diabetes), strict glycemic compensation is not required for diabetes patients with DFS. Increasing evidence indicates that intensive glycemic control delays the onset and slows the progression of diabetic retinopathy, nephropathy, and neuropathy in patients with insulin-dependent diabetes mellitus. Intensive glycemic control has to accompany careful monitoring – strict glycemic control can lead to profound hypoglycemia. Callaghan et al. performed a meta-analysis of the effect of intensive glycemic control on diabetic neuropathy and demonstrated a significantly reduced risk of developing clinical neuropathy with better glycemic control, especially in type 1 diabetes mellitus. Strict glycemic control is currently the only effective tool for preventing or delaying the development of neuropathy in patients with type 1 diabetes and slowing the progression of neuropathy in some patients with type 2 diabetes.

The basis of treatment is to modify lifestyle, maintain weight, increase physical activity, and reduce energy intake (fewer drinks and foods sweetened with sugar, reduce consumption of foods with a high-fat content).

In DM type 1, we start insulin treatment in an intensified regimen (basal + prandial insulin) with human insulins, possibly combined with insulin analogs or an intensified regimen with insulin analogs.

In DM type 2, metformin is the drug of choice. If the treatment is contraindicated or not tolerated by the patient, the following can be used: sulfonylurea derivatives, glitazones, and glinides. Sulfonylurea derivatives have a rapid onset of action. The most used are gliclazide MR and glimepiride due to the low incidence of hypoglycemia and minimal weight gain during treatment. Pioglitazone is the most widely used of the glitazones, and it can also be used in obese patients without heart failure. Glinides (repaglinide, nateglinide) are suitable for postprandial hyperglycemia due to their rapid onset of action.

Alpha-glucosidase inhibitors (acarbose) are suitable for patients with less pronounced fasting hyperglycemia and postprandial hyperglycemia.

DPP-4 inhibitors are used in combined treatment; they are weight-neutral, do not cause hypoglycemia, and have minimal side effects.

GLP-1 receptor antagonists are considered in obese patients.

The most common are combinations of all available antidiabetic drugs with metformin.

Management of associated risk factors

The associated risk factors are atherosclerosis and cardiovascular diseases. In patients with DFS, it is almost always advanced DM with chronic, manifesting complications. The basis is regime measures (diet, smoking ban, weight reduction). A 100 mg dose of ASA daily is recommended if cardiovascular diseases manifest (secondary prevention). A large percentage of diabetes patients have resistance to this active substance, therefore, the strict administration of ASA for all diabetes patients is waived. It is essential to maintain normotension in elderly diabetics up to 140/90 mm Hg. Arterial hypertension is primarily treated with ACE inhibitors or sartans. If they are ineffective, we add calcium channel blockers, beta-blockers, or diuretics. This is how we slow down the development of diabetic nephropathy, which we monitor using albuminuria. If there are elevated creatinine values, we consult a nephrologist. Dyslipidemia is treated by achieving a level of LDL cholesterol below 2.5 mmol/l, with the manifestation of cardiovascular disease below 1.8 mmol/l using statins. Statins reduce the incidence of cardiovascular events in diabetes patients. To intensify the treatment, we can combine them with omega-3 fatty acids. The secondary goal is to reduce the TAG level to 1.5 mmol/l and increase HDL cholesterol. To achieve that, we can use fibrates or a combination of hypolipidemic treatments.

Table 3.2 Risk stratification for assessing the risk of developing a diabetic foot or amputation (source: Department of Vascular Surgery VUSCH)

Low risk	Medium risk	High risk
risk factors are not present	deformities	previous ulcer
formation of one callus	neuropathy	amputation in the past
	absence of critical ischemia	treatment of renal insufficiency
		neuropathy and absence of critical ischemia
		neuropathy with callus and/or deformity
		absence of critical ischemia with callus and/or deformity

The DFS may not always have a bad prognosis; if a proper diagnosis is followed by adequate treatment, the condition may not result in amputation. It is reported that a modern, multidisciplinary approach can reduce amputations by 43-86%. In a patient with an open wound on the leg, the risk of re-ulceration is up to 50% within one year.

A critical component is patient compliance. It should be remembered that DFS is a serious complication of diabetes which most significantly interferes with the patient's mobility, negatively affecting his psyche.

Diagnosis of ischemic injury

It is again based on anamnesis, physical examination, and the following examination methods: positional and stress tests of the lower limbs (Prusík and Ratschow tests). The positional test has a phase of passive elevation of the lower limb (raised above the mat at a 45° angle for 30 seconds), an active phase (during elevation, the patient performs dorsiflexion and plantar flexion until pain occurs), and a hyperemia phase (the patient sits down and lowers lower limbs from the bed and we monitor the time of the first redness – the norm is within 5 seconds).

The primary non-invasive imaging method is duplex ultrasonography and the Doppler ultrasound meter, allowing us to determine the ankle-brachial index (ABI).

It indirectly indicates atherosclerotic involvement of the coronary, cerebral, and renal vessels. Since measuring distal pressures in people with

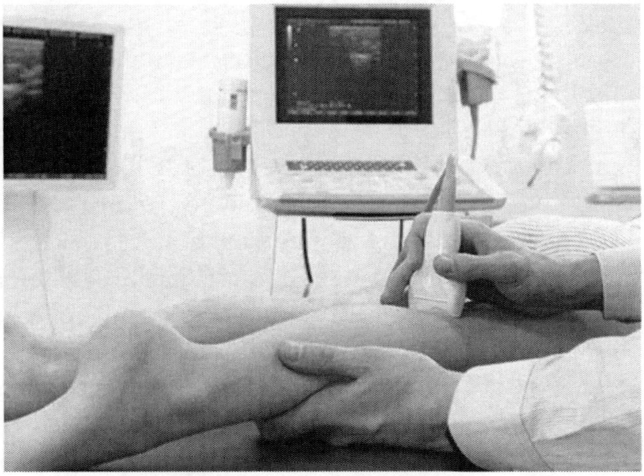

Figure 3.3 USG examination of the patient (source: Department of Vascular Surgery VUSCH).

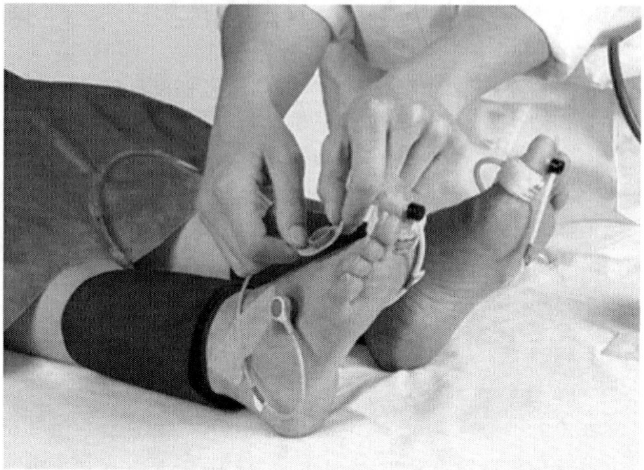

Figure 3.4 Transcutaneous oximetry in diabetic foot syndrome (source: Department of Vascular Surgery VUSCH).

diabetes fails due to the development of mediocalcinosis, measuring finger pressures with a special finger cuff is also used. Transcutaneous measuring of the partial pressure of oxygen (TcPO2) also appears to be a suitable method. Based on it, we evaluate the oxygenation of the tissues, which can be used to determine the level of the amputation. It was first used in 1978. It monitors the dependence of TcPO2 changes on arterial perfusion pressure, which affects TcPO2 in ischemic conditions.

In atherosclerosis, mainly large and medium limb arteries are obliterated; thus, the symptoms of tissue ischemia develop. An adequate partial pressure of oxygen is essential for hypoxic non-healing wounds, and the oxygen pressure is 5-15 mm Hg. A partial oxygen pressure of at least 30-40 mm Hg is necessary for fibroblastic proliferation, collagen synthesis, and capillary proliferation. It improves the bactericidal activity of leukocytes, which is a possible explanation for the beneficial effect of hyperbaric oxygen therapy. Most authors indicate that a stump after amputation of the lower leg heals primarily in 90% of cases, with TcPO2 values of more than 30-35 mm Hg measured approximately 10 cm below the knee. With lower pressure, it healed in only 66% of cases. An increase in the level of glycated hemoglobin can affect TcPO2 values. Hyperglycemia causes a change in the rheological properties of blood in people with diabetes, with a significant decrease in TcPO2 values. Several authors found that age, sex, and smoking did not have such an effect on TcPO2 as diabetes. TcPO2 examination is not affected by mediocalcinosis. However, it is significantly affected by inflammation. In the acute phase, the reduced pH value and inflammatory mediators cause arterioles and capillaries to dilate, reducing the blood flow rate depending on the perfusion pressure. Arteriovenous anastomoses open, and blood bypasses the cutaneous capillary plexus. Blood stasis occurs in the venules; the perfusion conditions deteriorate, and the venules and arterioles dilate, leading to endothelial dysfunction. Its permeability increases, and plasma proteins and fibrinogen escape; fibrin is deposited in the interstitium of blood vessels, which worsens tissue hypoxia and malnutrition in the surrounding area, which results macroscopically in trophic changes in the skin of the leg. Leukocytes accumulate in the interstitium, thus enhancing inflammatory processes. Histamine, kinins, and prostaglandins cause increased fluid losses into the interstitium. Oncotic pressure rises, and fluid reabsorption worsens, increasing oxygen diffusion distance. Infections and repair processes of the skin significantly increase oxygen consumption. The goal of surgeons when amputating a limb is to amputate it at the lowest possible level with the 'per primam' healing of the stump. In addition to the aforementioned, tissue hypoxia, infection, necrotic papules, poor treatment, a generally poor condition in connection with febrility, and malnutrition are important factors of poor wound healing. With TcPO2 values below 20 mm Hg, the probability of non-healing of the wound was 39 times higher than with standard values. Up to 50% of DFS patients suffer from mediocalcinosis, which occurs in 5-10% of people with diabetes. On physical examination, the arteries are stiff and incompressible; calcium salts are deposited in the artery wall. When measuring the systolic pressure by Doppler, false positive results are recorded.

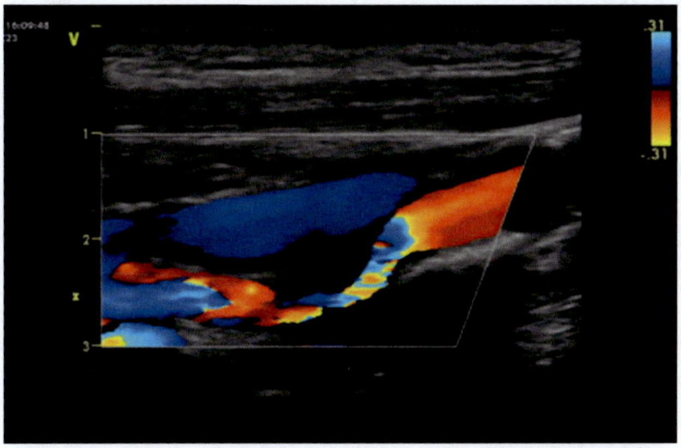

Figure 3.5 USG representation of superficial femoral artery (SFA) stenosis (source: Department of Vascular Surgery VUSCH).

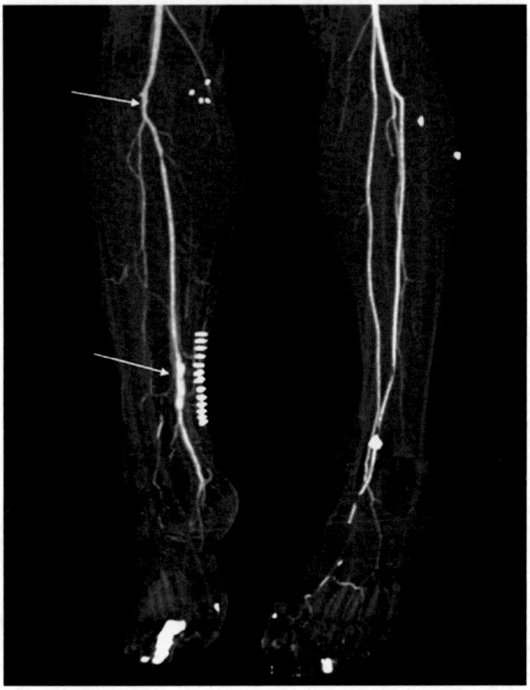

Figure 3.6 CT representation of stenosis of lower leg arteries (source: Department of Vascular Surgery VUSCH).

A "rail-like" strip of the tunica media is visible in the case of mediocalcinosis on X-ray images, in contrast to complicated atherosclerotic plaques, which appear as a spotted, interrupted pattern. Mediocalcinosis often coincides with autonomic neuropathy.

Computed tomography (CT) is rarely used in the diagnosis of DFS. It can show bone changes, skeleton destruction, periosteum reactions, bone gas bubbles, and sequestration. If a contrast agent is applied, it can visualize the arterial system.

Magnetic resonance imaging (MRI) is the dominant method in diagnosing complicated DFS. Thanks to its distinguishing ability, it can localize neuropathy and distinguish it from the inflammation of soft tissues. However, it cannot differentiate the early stages of osteomyelitis and osteoarthropathy, but it is the primary method in diagnosing Charcot neuropathic osteoarthropathy.

Diagnostic angiography

It is the "gold standard" of arterial imaging. It is performed by retrograde puncture of the common femoral artery so that the area from the abdominal

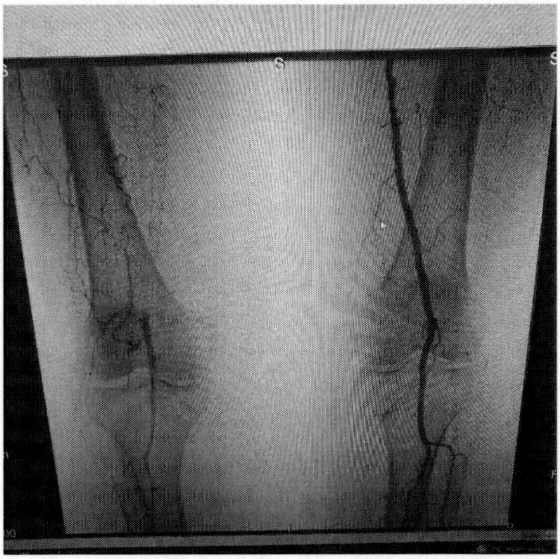

Figure 3.7 Diagnostic angiography (arteries of the right lower limb - source: Department of Vascular Surgery VUSCH).

aorta, pelvic arteries, and lower limbs will be displayed. Based on the result, the following therapeutic procedure will be decided (endovascular solution vs. angiosurgical revascularization). Imaging methods aim to show and correctly interpret the changes in the affected leg, which can be challenging because there is a combination of pathological processes in the diabetic leg.

CT angiography (CTA) partially replaces DSA, mainly thanks to multi-detector devices and the possibility of data reconstruction into 2D and 3D images. The examination takes less time; it can also be performed outpatient, and the contrast material is administered intravenously. When imaging peripheral arteries (distal from the knee), DSA is more accurate, especially in people with diabetes. Artifacts in the venous filling impair the evaluation of the arteries, and the image quality is worse in patients with lower cardiac output. Another disadvantage is that more contrast material needs to be administered.

MR angiography (MRA) is relatively accurate in imaging and quantifying calcified stenoses; however, like CTA, it cannot accurately image damage to the crural arteries. The disadvantages are also poorer availability, higher price, and demands for patient cooperation, especially if they have an implanted pacemaker. However, it can also be used to examine patients with an allergy to iodine and renal insufficiency.

Other imaging methods in diabetic foot syndrome

One of the primary imaging methods is an X-ray image. It is always available and relatively cheap. On the X-ray image, we can observe the signs of osteomyelitis and osteoarthropathy. However, it will not show osteomyelitis in the initial stages (up to 14 days). Changes are typically localized in the front part of the foot (phalanges, metatarsal heads, calcaneus area). In the early stages, cortical erosions, periostoses, lytic defects on the cortex, pyarthrosis (widening of the joint space), gas, osteoporotic changes, defects of soft parts, and edema are visible in the image. These abnormalities appear with a 7-15 day delay from the onset of clinical symptoms of acute osteomyelitis, so it is diagnostically challenging to differentiate them in time. Therefore, in the first weeks of the development of the disease, the picture is negative. Consequently, it is necessary to repeat the image after 7-14 days. If the skeleton remains intact, the infection spreads in the soft tissues. If the finding is unclear or ambiguous, other diagnostic options should be continued (MRI, scintigraphy of the skeleton, scintigraphy with labeled leukocytes). In the chronic stage of osteomyelitis, the bone is sclerotic, mottled, saturated, loses its structure, the medullary cavity disappears, and ankylosis of the joints and deformity of the leg is visible.

Scintigraphy

It shows functional and metabolic changes in tissues. The image is created by ionizing radiation emanating from the patient's body. The source is a radiopharmaceutical. The most frequently used radionuclide is 99mTc. It is a pure gamma emitter with a short half-life. The advantage is the low dose absorbed in the patient's body. The disadvantage is the poorer spatial resolution and, thus, poorer determination of the exact location of the radiopharmaceutical accumulation.

With scintigraphy of the skeleton, we can detect changes associated with osteomyelitis already 24 hours after the onset of inflammation. Yet, still, we cannot determine the differences between infectious and non-infectious inflammation. Diagnostics uses pathophysiological changes during inflammation. Phosphonates labeled with 99mTc are administered intravenously and monitored with a gamma camera in three/four phases. In the first three phases, we observe increased blood flow, asymmetric tissue perfusion, and bone remodeling. To distinguish osteomyelitis from cellulitis, a fourth phase is often necessary, which is done after 24 hours. In osteomyelitis, the radiopharmaceutical accumulation is high; on the contrary, it decreases in cellulitis.

Scintigraphy with labeled leukocytes uses their 99 mTc labeling and their accumulation at the site of inflammation. However, the sensitivity is low in chronic inflammations. However, it can help differentiate between osteomyelitis and Charcot osteoarthropathy. Leukocyte accumulation after 4 and 24 hours is compared. While in osteoarthropathy, the accumulation decreases, in osteomyelitis, it is constant or rises. If, for example, the increased accumulation of labeled leukocytes persists after 3-4 weeks of antibiotic treatment, there is a high probability of amputation. The last step in diagnosis is a bone biopsy, where a sample is taken either through a puncture or an open route. However, with long-term antibiotic treatment, the sample can already be sterile.

If we summarize the given imaging methods, the first choice is an X-ray image of the foot in two projections. Suppose the X-ray finding is repeatedly negative, and it is a patient without a defect with clinically proven neuropathy. In that case, we perform CT, which will also show neuropathic changes that the X-ray image does not show. In case of suspicion of infection, we add bone scintigraphy and an MRI examination. When using MRI with contrast, we will also show the extent of soft tissue infection (ischemia, necrosis), which helps in planning the surgical treatment of the defect. The availability of these modalities, the quality of the equipment, the experience of the staff, and the correct technical execution of the examination and, above all, its proper interpretation are essential.

In patients in stage III and stage IV of PAD (according to Fontain), in patients with CLI (pain at rest, non-healing defects of lower limbs), we indicate an angiographic examination to determine the anatomical localization of the disease and to choose the most appropriate treatment method (endovascular vs. angiosurgical). When confirming atherosclerotic PAD, we screen the carotid, coronary, renal, and abdominal aorta areas. During five years, out of 100 patients suffering from claudication, 30 died, 16 of them due to acute myocardial infarction, and four died due to cerebrovascular causes.

The treatment of diabetic ulcers represents a growing socio-economic burden, with an estimated cost of £580 million in 2010–2011 in the UK, of which more than half was spent on diabetic foot care. It is obvious that the later stages of diabetic foot are associated with severe morbidity and an overall reduction in quality of life.

References

Andersen H. Motor dysfunction in diabetes. Diabet. Metab. Res. Rev. 2012;28:89–92. DOI: 10.1002/dmrr.2257.

Boucek P. Advanced diabetic neuropathy—A point of no return? Rev. Diabet. Stud. 2006;3:143–150. DOI 10.1900/RDS.2006.3.143.

Boulton A.J. Diabetic neuropathy and foot complications. Handbook Clin. Neurol. 2014;126:97–107.

Boulton A.J. The diabetic foot: Grand overview, epidemiology, and pathogenesis. Diabet./Metab. Res. Rev. 2008;24:S3–S6.

Boulton A.J. The pathway to foot ulceration in diabetes. Med. Clin. N. Am. 2013;97:775–790. DOI: 10.1016/j.mcna.2013.03.007.

Boulton A.J. What you can't feel can hurt you. J. Vasc. Surg. 2010;52:28S–30S. DOI: 10.1016/j.jvs.2010.06.005.

Boulton A.J., Kirsner R.S., Vileikyte L. Clinical practice. Neuropathic diabetic foot ulcers. N. Engl. J. Med. 2004;351:48–55. DOI: 10.1056/NEJMcp032966.

Brandner J.M., Zacheja S., Houdek P., Moii I., Lobmann R. Expression of matrix metalloproteinases, cytokines, and connexins in diabetic and nondiabetic human keratinocytes before and after transplantation into an ex vivo wound-healing model. Diabet. Care. 2008;31:114–120. DOI: 10.2337/dc07-1304.

Bruhn-Olszewska B., Korzon-Burakowska A., Gabig-Ciminska M., Olszewski P., Wegrzyn A., Jakobkiewicz-Banecka J. Molecular factors involved in the development of diabetic foot syndrome. Acta Biochim. Pol. 2012;59:507–513.

Da Silva L., Carvalho E., Cruz M.T. Role of neuropeptides in skin inflammation and its involvement in diabetic wound healing. Exp. Opin. Biol. Ther. 2010;10:1427–1439. DOI: 10.1517/14712598.2010.515207.

Gilbey S.G. Neuropathy and foot problems in diabetes. Clin. Med. 2004;4:318–323. DOI: 10.7861/clinmedicine.4-4-318

Kamenov Z.A., Traykov L.D. Diabetic autonomic neuropathy. Adv. Exp. Med. Biol. 2012;771:176–193.

Kamenov Z.A., Traykov L.D. Diabetic somatic neuropathy. Adv. Exp. Med. Biol. 2012;771:155–175.

Krahulec B. et al.: Manažment pacienta so syndrómom diabetickej nohy. VEDA, 2013; s.85–93.

Lobmann R. Diabetic foot syndrome. Der Internist. 2011;52:539–548. doi: 10.1007/s00108-010-2733.

Lobmann R. Diabetic foot: How to avoid therapeutic mistakes. MMW Fortschr. Der Med. 2013;155:63–66. DOI: 10.1007/s15006-013-2284.

Lobmann R., Ambrosch A., Schultz G., Waldmann K., Schiweck S., Lehnert H. Expression of matrix-metalloproteinases and their inhibitors in the wounds of diabetic and non-diabetic patients. Diabetologia. 2002;45:1011–1016. DOI: 10.1007/s00125-002-0868-8.

Molines L., Darmon P., Raccah D. Charcot's foot: Newest findings on its pathophysiology, diagnosis, and treatment. Diabet. Metab. 2010;36:251–255. DOI: 10.1016/j.diabet.2010.04.002.

Monteiro-Soares M., Boyko E.J., Ribeiro J., Dinis-Ribeiro L.M. Risk stratification systems for diabetic foot ulcers: A systematic review. Diabetologia. 2011;54:1190–1199. DOI: 10.1007/s00125-010-2030-3.

Peltier A., Goutman S.A., Callaghan B.C. Painful diabetic neuropathy. BMJ. 2014;348:g1799. DOI: 10.1136/BMJ.g1799.

Risse A. Syndróm diabetickej nohy – interdisciplinárna výzva. Hamostaseológia. 2007; 27 :117-122.

Rumenapf G., Dittler S., Morbach S., Amendt K., Radu A. The vascular surgeon's role in interdisciplinary treatment of diabetic foot syndrome. Der Chir. Z. Fuer Alle Geb. Der Oper. Med. 2008;79:535–545.

Russell J.W., Zilliox L.A. Diabetic neuropathies. Continuum. 2014;20:1226–1240. DOI: 10.1212/01.CON.0000455884.29545.d2.

Said G. Diabetic neuropathy. Handbook Clin. Neurol. 2013;115:579–589.

Sandireddy R., Yerra V.G., Areti A., Komirishetty P., Kumar A. Neuroinflammation and oxidative stress in diabetic neuropathy: Futuristic strategies based on these targets. Int. J. Endocrinol. 2014;2014:674987. DOI: 10.1155/2014/674987.

Singh V.P., Bali A., Singh N., Jaggi A.S. Advanced glycation end products and diabetic complications. Korean J. Physiol. Pharmacol. 2014;18:1–14. DOI: 10.4196/kjpp.2014.18.1.1. [PMC free article] [PubMed] [CrossRef] [Google Scholar]

Tavee J., Zhou L. Small fiber neuropathy: A burning problem. Clevel. Clin. J. Med. 2009;76:297–305. DOI: 10.3949/ccjm.76a.08070.

Van Battum P., Schaper N., Prompers L., Apelqvist J., Jude E. Differences in minor amputation rate in diabetic foot disease throughout Europe are in part explained by differences in disease severity at presentation. Diabet. Med. J. Br. Diabet. Assoc. 2011;28:199–205.

Vinik A.I., Maser R.E., Mitchell B.D., Freeman R. Diabetic autonomic neuropathy. Diabet.Care. 2003;26:1553–1579. DOI: 10.2337/diacare.26.5.1553.

Zenker J., Ziegler D., Chrast R. Novel pathogenic pathways in diabetic neuropathy. Trends Neurosci. 2013;36:439–449. DOI: 10.1016/j.tins.2013.04.008.

Ziegler D., Keller J., Maier C., Pannek J. Diabetic neuropathy. Exp. Clin. Endocrinol. Diabet. Off. J. Ger. Soc. Endocrinol. Ger. Diabet. Assoc. 2014;122:406–415.

Zimmermann A., Reeps C., Hartl F., Ockert S., Eckstein H.H. The diabetic foot. Der Chir. Z. Fuer Alle Geb. Der Oper. Med. 2009;80:430–436.

Chapter 4

Classification and Treatment of Diabetic Foot Infections

Martina Zavacká, MD*

Department of Vascular Surgery, East Slovak Institute of Cardiovascular Diseases, Faculty of Medicine, Pavol Jozef Šafárik University in Košice, Slovakia

Abstract

Diabetic foot syndrome is defined by the WHO as ulceration and destruction of leg tissue associated with neuropathy, angiopathy, and infection. Due to its frequent relapses, it is considered lifelong. It is one of the most severe complications of diabetes. It is a frequent cause of hospitalization and disability of people with diabetes. There are various classification scales, e.g., the clinical Wagner classification of the diabetic foot, based on assessing the presence of infection and depth of ulceration. Comprehensive prevention and therapy of diabetic legs can reduce the number of amputations by 50% and can significantly reduce the cost of long-term treatment.

Key Words: diabetic foot syndrome, angiopathy, neuropathy, disability, diabetes mellitus, ulcerations

Introduction

The WHO defines diabetic foot syndrome as 'ulceration and destruction of foot tissue associated with neuropathy, angiopathy, and infection.' Because of its frequent recurrences, it is considered lifelong. It is one of the most severe complications of diabetes: approximately 50% of all non-traumatic amputations

* Corresponding Author's Email: martina.zavacka@upjs.sk

In: Diabetic Foot
Editor: Martina Zavacká
ISBN: 979-8-89113-019-7

are performed in patients with diabetes. It is also a frequent cause of hospitalization and disability for people with diabetes.

Risk factors for ulceration are previous ulcerations or amputations, sensorimotor neuropathy, injuries (due to falls, walking barefoot, inappropriate footwear), biomechanical factors (reduced joint mobility, leg deformities, hyperkeratosis), ischemic disease of the lower limbs, social and economic factors (low social status, insufficient health care).

Classification of diabetic foot syndrome

Different scales are used for classification, e.g., the clinical classification of the diabetic foot according to Wagner, which is based on the assessment of the presence of infection and the depth of ulceration:

Grade 0: high risk of ulceration
Grade 1: superficial ulcerations in the skin not exceeding the subcutaneous fat layer
Grade 2: deeper ulcerations that extend beyond the subcutaneous fat layer and spread to joint capsules, tendons, or bones without signs of deep infection.
Grade 3: deep infection (e.g., abscess, tendinitis, arthritis, etc.). This condition threatens the patient's limb and requires hospitalization and surgical treatment, which in most cases can be done without amputation.
Grade 4: localized gangrene, which most often affects the fingers, heel, or front part of the leg. At this stage, saving the limb and preventing amputation is still possible.
Grade 5: extensive gangrene or necrosis stage, which already requires amputation.

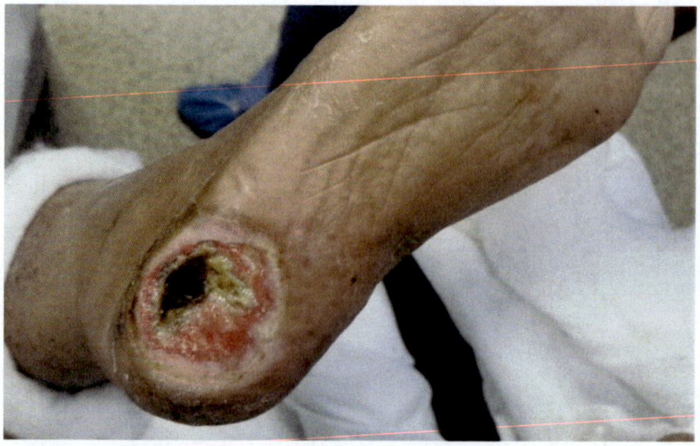

Figure 4.1 Patient with diabetic foot (source: Department of Vascular Surgery VUSCH).

Grade 0

The leg has an intact skin cover. There are no open lesions present. The appearance of the leg can vary: from a well-hydrated, healthy leg to a dystrophic leg with numerous bony deformities, a non-palpable pulse, to a partially amputated leg with no signs of ulcerations. The feet of diabetics in the early stage of the disease still have preserved sensitivity and react to infection or injury like in non-diabetics. With the gradual development of the disease, the vascular and neurological condition of the patient worsens. Therefore, it is unusual to encounter patients with long-lasting diabetes without evidence of neuropathy (Melton et al., 1980). Neuropathy of the intrinsic muscles of the feet leads to contracture and deviation of the toes. Vascular disorders are two to three times more common in patients with neuropathy. The primary therapeutic goal of grade zero is a conservative approach. Regular podiatric check-ups are recommended for patients. Palliative debridement of hyperkeratotic lesions, dystrophic and onychomycosis toenails should not be underestimated. We analyze the biomechanics of walking in the patient to balance the feet and redistribute the body weight to ensure the longevity of the tissue in the pressure points. Prosthetic aids are essential for correcting problematic types of walking. When proprioception deteriorates, Charcot changes begin to appear on the joints. In such cases, patients should wear custom-made shoes. Due to hereditary predisposition and imbalance of the internal muscles of the foot associated with diabetes, patients often experience ingrown toenails, hammer toes, hallux valgus, and exostoses on feet. Since these deformities lead to a violation of the skin cover, preventive surgical intervention should be considered. Later, the condition worsens, and the risk of surgery increases. If the leg is ischemic, podiatric surgery should be considered only after successful revascularization. With an ankle-brachial index of 0.70 and above, we assume the possibility of healing the defect. The goal of diabetic foot care is to maintain a grade 0 for as long as possible.

Grade 1

It is characterized by a superficial ulcer that does not penetrate the entire dermis but is not infected. We distinguish two types of ulcers: ischemic and neuropathic. Appearance and management vary. Ischemic ulcers occur anywhere on the leg but are highly resistant to treatment. No significant hyperkeratosis is usually present. These lesions are painful and quickly become infected if not treated early. The debridement of the ischemic lesion uncovers the deeper fibrotic ischemic tissue. A neuropathic ulcer is associated with persistent pressure. In contrast, these lesions are painless, and hyperkeratosis is generally present. Debridement is necessary for granulations and epithelialization.

The distribution of weight forces is important. Unless the uncontrolled infection is present, neurotrophic lesions have a good prognosis for healing.

Grade 2

There is a deeply infected ulcer, often uncovering a bone or tendon. Debridement and drainage of abscesses should be performed as soon as possible. We always take samples for cultivation and deploy antibiotic treatment. The only contraindication to debridement and drainage of the infected ulcer is gangrene or an extensive infection that requires amputation as a first choice. If the lesion is ischemic, a vascular examination is necessary to evaluate the need for revascularization. During the entire management of this condition, it should be borne in mind that diabetic infection is unstable and can quickly shift from a controlled to a fulminant type of infection. Although anatomical structures near the superficial transverse ligament form natural barriers against infection, subtle infectious diabetic microangiopathy can breach these anatomical barriers and allow infection to spread along structures that would typically stop the spread of infection. In addition to the narrowing of blood vessels, diabetes is also associated with other microcirculatory abnormalities: reduced flexibility of red blood cells and increased blood viscosity. Acute thrombotic occlusion of blood vessels at the site of infection is common. After managing the infection, the tissues are recanalized and granulated. In diabetics, the vascular predisposition may accentuate the occlusion so that the infection may spread to the ever-enlarging areas of necrosis. When the terminal artery is occluded, the tissue supplied by it becomes necrotic.

Charcot osteoarthropathy is a progressive, painless, destructive process primarily involving the foot and ankle. It is created due to a neurotraumatic and neurovascular combination that leads to fracture or joint damage. Culture from bone is necessary for the differential diagnosis. If osteomyelitis is detected, this condition must be dealt with vigorously. If Charcot osteoarthrosis is diagnosed, ostectomy or joint fusion should be considered after controlling the infection. With conservative treatment, ulcers of the second degree can be closed. If the conservative treatment proves ineffective, bone excision and graft application should be considered to achieve closure of the defect.

Grade 3

It is distinguished from Grade 2 by localized cellulitis, swelling, and hyperemia. Grade 3 diabetic foot infection may include fascial infection, deep abscess, and septic impairment down to the bone level, causing necrotizing fasciitis, osteomyelitis, gas gangrene, and necrotizing cellulitis. Hospitalization is indicated with parenteral administration of antibiotics and X-ray examination to rule out bone impairment or the presence of gas in soft tissues. We perform drainage and debridement of ischemic tissue as soon as possible and collect material for culture. Parenteral antibiotic treatment is continued until the culture results are negative and the laboratory parameters are normal. The wound usually heals secondarily. Caring for a grade 3 diabetic foot requires a coordinated effort by the healthcare team aiming to return the foot to grade 0.

Grade 4

It includes gangrene of the forefoot. Its presence requires amputation of the affected body part at the appropriate level. Every effort should be made to save as much of the still functional leg as possible. The chances of salvaging the grade 4 diabetic foot are significantly reduced due to vascular insufficiency. The risk of failure is high, so amputation is often approached at a higher level. Revascularization before the procedure can reduce the height of the amputation.

Grade 5

The diabetic foot is gangrenous and requires amputation at ankle level or higher. Patients with sufficient vascular supply with gangrene only in the front part of the foot are possible candidates for Syme's amputation or exarticulation at the ankle level. Other patients require amputation at the below knee or thigh level. Due to the high mortality rate after amputation, strict care by a diabetologist is necessary. Rehabilitation and training in walking with a prosthesis should be indicated as soon as possible.

Other types of diabetic foot classifications

Texas classification (University of Texas Wound Classification System).

In this classification, four grades of disability are distinguished: 0, I, II, and III. Lesions are graded according to the depth of ulceration.

Grade 0 – pre-ulcerous or post-ulcerous condition with complete ulceration.
Grade I. a superficial wound.
Grade II. a wound that affects the tendon or tendon sheath.
Grade III.- the wound extends to the bone or joint.

Each grade is complemented by a stage and has its own characteristics:

stage A (without infection and ischemia),
stage B (with infection),
stage C (with ischemia),
stage D (with infection and ischemia).

The depth of the ulceration is evaluated with the probe used to determine the superficial or deep wound and where it penetrates (tendons, joints, and bones).

The degree of infection is evaluated according to clinical signs, such as purulent secretion, increased body temperature, pain, redness, dysfunction, etc.

The extent of ischemia is evaluated according to clinical and non-invasive examination (peripheral pulsation and ankle-brachial index).

The S(AD) SAD classification proposed by MacFarlane and Jeffcoate evaluates:

Size(Area and Depth), Sepsis, Arteriopathy, and Denervation.

The previous classification complements and evaluates the degrees of neuropathy, angiopathy, and infection. It also assesses the depth and degree of ulceration.

PEDIS system divides ulcerations into five categories:

P – perfusion, E – extension, D – depth, I – infection, S – sensation. It is the most accurate classification system of those above, but it is used in international studies rather than in routine clinical practice (Jirkovská, 2006).

The importance of diabetic foot care is even more significant because the number of diabetic patients is increasing with life prolongation due to current medical advances. Unfortunately, the tendency to affect the limb also increases with age. Despite significant improvements in healthcare for diabetic patients, their neurotrophic and vascular problems persist.

The latest classification of ulcerations was created according to the international consensus in 2003 to accurately characterize wounds so that they are comparable in the healing assessment.

It evaluates:

a) 3 stages of tissue perfusion,
b) wound size in cm2,
c) 3 degrees of the depth of the wound,
d) 4 stages of infection,
e) 2 degrees of sensitivity.

The international consensus of the diabetic foot syndrome indicates these risk factors: previous amputation and ulceration of the foot, sensory-motor neuropathy, trauma (walking barefoot, inappropriate shoes, small objects in shoes, accidents, and falls), deformities and hyperkeratosis of the foot, ischemic disease of the lower limbs, socio-economic factors (patient's unwillingness to cooperate, poor availability of podiatric care).

A large number of factors and disorders related to diabetes directly or indirectly contribute to defect formation (e.g., neuropathy, ischemic disease of the lower limbs, smoking, early infection, phlegmons, abscesses, purulent arthritis, osteomyelitis), severe deformities (Charcot's osteoarthropathy), joint mobility disorders, hyperkeratosis, edema, and acquired immune disorders. The primary care for patients with diabetic foot syndrome is a systematic education of the patient, early diagnosis, and an effort for causal therapy of the ulceration.

Foot infections are common in diabetic patients. They are the leading cause of hospitalization and amputation of the lower limbs. Aggressive and urgent surgical intervention is necessary for life- or limb-threatening infection to save and salvage the limb. Critical limb ischemia and neuropathy complicate the treatment of severe diabetic foot infection. It carries a 25% risk of above-knee amputation. The overall strategy for surgical management of severe diabetic foot infection is as follows: the first step is to control the infection through extensive surgical debridement, the second step is a comprehensive examination of the vessels with possible vascular surgery and/or endovascular intervention, and the last step is soft tissue and skeletal reconstruction after eradication of the infection, to achieve the wound closure and saving of the limb. A consistent step-by-step surgical approach and sound principles are paramount to successfully managing a severe diabetic foot infection. Proper timing and execution will reduce mortality, morbidity, psychological distress, and length of hospitalization associated with life- or limb-threatening infections.

Infectious complications of the diabetic foot are a frequent reason for hospitalization of people with diabetes. As a cause of diabetic ulceration, they play a less important role (less than 1% of cases). However, as a risk factor for future amputation, the role of infection is gaining importance. It is necessary to realize that infectious complications in diabetics may not be manifested by classic clinical or laboratory signs of inflammation, but hyperglycemia is often present. According to the depth of impact, a distinction is made between superficial and deep infection. According to the degree of severity of the clinical picture, a distinction is made between infections that do not threaten the limb (associated with superficial cellulitis around the wound up to 2 cm, without systemic symptoms, can be treated in outpatient conditions), infections that threaten the limb (cellulitis of a greater extent than 2 cm associated with lymphangitis, abscess, and osteomyelitis, requiring hospitalization) and life-threatening infections. A single type of microbe usually causes superficial infections; deep infections are polymicrobial. Two-thirds of the most common bacteria found in diabetic foot infections are staphylococci; then, it is streptococci, Pseudomonas aeruginosa, Proteus, Klebsiella, E. coli, and anaerobes, including Bacteroides, Clostridium, and Peptostreptococcus. A severe problem in diabetes patients is the development of osteomyelitis. Approximately 60% of ulcerations that do not heal are complicated by osteomyelitis, which results from the spread of infection from the skin's surface layers through the soft tissues to the bone. The process can affect any bone on the leg, but the metatarsal heads and toes are most often affected. In clinical practice, a frequent problem is a differential diagnosis of Charcot osteoarthropathy. However, this differentiation is necessary for the following therapeutic procedure. While massive long-term antibiotic treatment with possible surgical intervention up to the amputation is required in the case of infectious disease, in osteoarthropathy, a conservative approach with long-term limb immobilization and medical treatment prevails.

Osteomyelitis is probable in case of ulceration and positivity of 3 of these criteria:

1. the presence of phlegmon
2. probe-to-bone test at the base of ulceration
3. positive bacteriological findings from deep tissues
4. radiological and/or scintigraphy signs of osteitis
5. histological diagnosis.

A bone biopsy is considered the reference method for the diagnosis of osteomyelitis, but after antibiotics treatment, a false negative result can be obtained. Treatment: Broad-spectrum antibiotics are used, preferably according to culture and sensitivity. It is advisable to apply prophylactic treatment in case of deeper ulcerations, even in the case of a negative culture, because

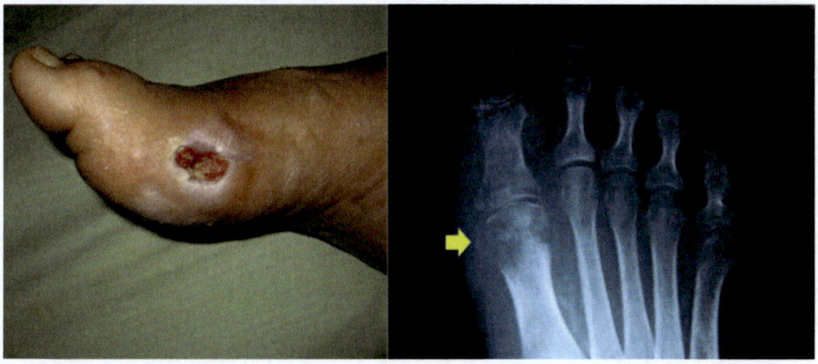

Figure 4.2 Clinical and X-ray correlation of osteomyelitis in diabetic foot syndrome (source: Department of Vascular Surgery VUSCH).

the infection often resides in deeper structures and may not be caught with a routine swab.

Diagnostic process

Clinical examination specifies the depth and extent of the defect. The infection may initially appear as cellulitis. An abscess (gangrene) may develop from it. It is essential to monitor elevated body temperature and laboratory elevation of C-reactive protein associated with leukocytosis. Microorganisms responsible for the infection should be isolated and identified from the bacteriological sample. Contamination with normal flora that colonizes the skin should be avoided. Before taking any sample, it is necessary to prepare the wound. A superficial wound swab is the most used method because it is the easiest. Deep swabbing and curettage of the ulcer can be performed using a curette or a sterile scalpel. A tissue biopsy is often made possible by neuropathy. Fine needle aspiration is a suitable method for sampling from deep wounds. Repetition is also recommended.

Radiological evaluation

An X-ray of the leg is performed primarily to check for signs of osteomyelitis or arthritis. Signs suggestive of a deep penetrating wound include periosteal reaction, osteopenia, and osteolysis. However, these symptoms only become apparent after 30-50% of the bone has been destroyed. At the beginning of the progression, X-ray plates may be normal. Therefore, they must be repeated every 2-4 weeks.

Echo Doppler and systolic pressure index (SPI) measurement

SPI measurement is a standard method of examination. It is performed using a continuous-wave Doppler probe. It corresponds to the ratio between the systolic pressure measured at the ankle in mmHg and the systolic pressure at the arm. An index between 0.7 and 0.9 indicates compensated PAD, while a value of less than 0.5 manifests severe ischemia. An SPI greater than 1.4 means that the distal arteries are calcified and incompressible (mediocalcinosis seen in 30% of diabetes patients).

Transcutaneous measurement of the partial pressure of oxygen (TcPO2)

It is an indirect measure to quantify the severity of skin ischemia. The obtained pressure value is an indicator of oxygenation of the surface layer of the skin. It reflects the nutritional efficiency of the microcirculation. It is a simple, non-invasive, and repeatable method, even in the case of mediocalcinosis. It is measured on the back of the foot and the first interosseous space. The normal TcPO 2 for a diabetic patient is around 50 mmHg.

TcPO 2 less than 35 mmHg manifests hypoxia at rest, indicating non-healing wounds. A measurement of <10 mmHg suggests the impossibility of healing, as the viability of the tissue is completely compromised. However, infection and edema of the hindfoot lead to falsely lower results.

Other examinations: measurement of systolic pressure on the big toe

The importance of this measurement in diabetes patients lies in the lower frequency of mediocalcinosis at the toe level. It is indicated in neuropathy cases accompanied by mediocalcinosis with ABI >1.4. There is a fully automatic and easy-to-use photoplethysmography in the evaluation process. Systolic pressure on the big toe higher than 30 mmHg shows an increased tendency to heal the ulcer. Ischemia is critical at values lower than 30 mmHg, and revascularization should be considered.

The statistical data of the National Center for Health Information for 2017 show that 6.78% of the population, i.e., almost every 15th Slovak, suffers from diabetes mellitus (DM). It is generally known that infectious diseases are more common in diabetics. It logically follows that examining biological material from patients diagnosed with diabetes mellitus should be routine in microbiological laboratories. Susceptibility to infections in people with diabetes mostly correlates with DM compensation, functional and structural organ changes, and patient age. These changes induce a reduced immune system activity and susceptibility to infections. Infections in diabetics have the same symptomatology as in patients without diabetes, but diabetics can be much more often affected by severe, even life-threatening complications.

Infections in diabetic patients can be classified as follows:

- **Infections associated with DM**
    - malignant otitis externa,
    - emphysematous pyelonephritis,
    - emphysematous cholecystitis,
    - mucormycosis.
- **Infections that occur more frequently in DM patients**
    - urinary tract infections (pyelonephritis, papillary necrosis, and others),
    - pulmonary complications of diabetes,
    - yeast diseases,
    - infections of soft tissues, fascia, and bones,
    - nosocomial infections,
    - sepsis.

In clinical practice, many wounds heal slowly and are difficult to treat. The recently introduced local topical negative pressure therapy (TNP) technique was developed to overcome some of these difficulties. TNP applies controlled negative pressure to the wound surface, which has potential advantages in wound treatment and management. Although the concept of using suction in wound treatment is familiar, applying negative pressure to the wound surface is new.

Wound treatment aims to create an environment that promotes healing or allows surgical intervention to cover and close the wound. The ideal internal environment for wound healing, as proposed by Winter, is moist (but not wet), non-infected, well-supplied with blood, and containing the right balance of inflammatory mediators. As a result, research has developed several dressings and treatment options, from simple gauze dressings to more complex

Table 4.1 Organ system, type of infection, and the most probable pathogen (Rybka, 2007)

Organ system	Type of infection	The most probable pathogen
respiratory tract	Community-acquired pneumonia	Staphylococcus aureus
		Streptococcus pneumoniae
		Klebsiella pneumoniae
		Legionella
	tuberculosis	Mycobacterium tuberculosis
	influenza	H1N1
urogenital tract	asymptomatic bacteriuria	E.coli
	cystitis	E.coli
		Acinetobacter
		Pseudomonas aeruginosa
		Group B streptococci
		Candida albicans
	perinephric abscess	E.coli
		enterobacteria
	pyelonephritis	E.coli
		Enterobacteria
		Proteus
		Klebsiella
gastrointestinal tract	oral and esophageal candidiasis	Candida albicans
	emphysematous cholecystitis	Clostridium perfringens
		E.coli
		Bacillus fragilis
	liver abscess	Klebsiella pneumoniae
skin and soft tissues	folliculitis	Group A Streptococci
		Staphylococcus aureus
	furunculosis	Streptococcus pneumoniae
	necrotic fasciitis	streptococci
		enterobacteria
	diabetic foot	Group A streptococci
		Staphylococcus aureus
		anaerobes
	otitis externa	Pseudomonas aeruginosa
		Aspergillus species
	Fournier gangrene	E.coli
		staphylococci
		streptococci
		Proteus
		Pseudomonas
		Clostridium perfringens

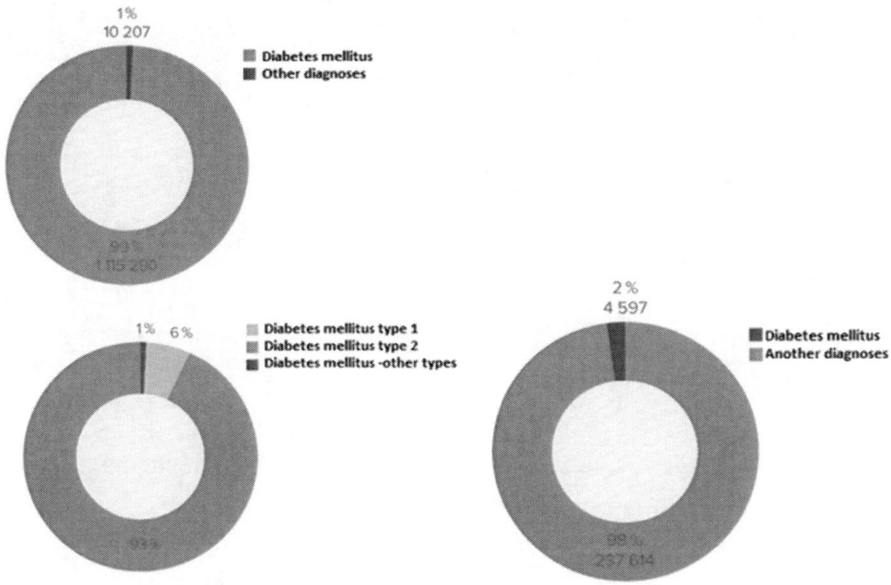

Figure 4.3 Statistics (source: www.nczi.sk).

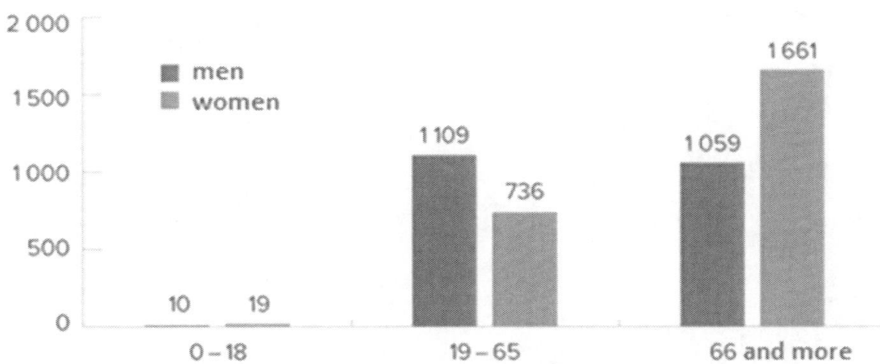

Figure 4.4 Statistics (source: www.nczi.sk).

chemical-impregnated dressings. In fact, special dressings are now available for specific types of wounds (e.g., moist, dry, dirty, exudate). This is often confusing and makes it difficult for many doctors to choose a dressing or treatment.

The concept of using negative pressure to create suction to allow drainage of surgical wounds to promote wound healing is well known. If excess fluid is not sufficiently removed from the wound after surgery, its components can serve as physical and chemical deterrents to wound healing. In practice,

Dg. Diabetes mellitus								
Age	GIT	lower respira-tory tract	GYN	upper respira-tory tract	hemo-cultures	Clinical	Urine	Total no. of positive results
0 – 18	2			13		1	13	29
19 – 65	9	96	19	212	43	1 051	418	1 848
66 and more	9	144	12	382	75	1 170	928	2 720
Total no. of positive results	20	240	31	607	118	2 222	1 359	4 597

Clinical samples		
Material	Number	%
Wound swab	1 393	62,69
Skin smear	213	9,58
Cannula	213	9,58
Different material	173	7,78
Buccal smear	111	4,99
Tip	46	2,07
Decubitus	25	1,12
Pus	15	0,67
Other clinical sample	33	1,48

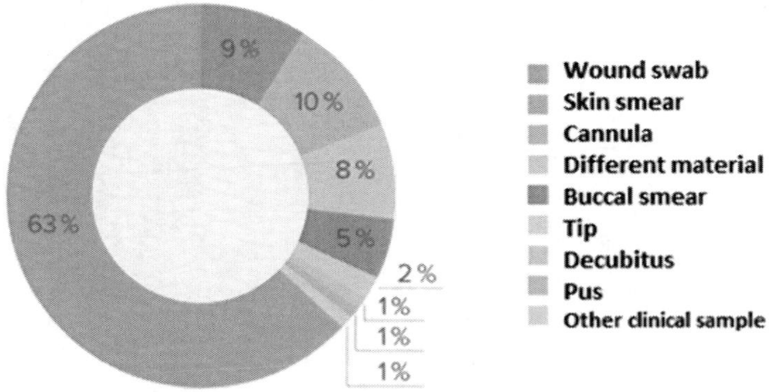

Figure 4.5 Statistics of diseases and clinical samples (source: www.nczi.sk).

it has been shown that the TNP therapy technique removes excess interstitial fluid and transfers mechanical force to the surrounding tissues, resulting in the deformation of the extracellular matrix and promoting wound size reduction.

Argenta and Morykwas published experimental work on TNP therapy first time in 1997 using animal and scientific studies. Using an acute wound model in pigs, Morykwas hypothesized a multimodal mechanism of action. Since then, the improved outcome parameters have been observed clinically in various wounds. This led to the widespread empirical acceptance of TNP and acted as a catalyst for developing several research programs.

TNP therapeutic equipment consists of a mesh foam dressing inserted into the wound and sealed with an adhesive bandage. Then, a suction force is applied through the wound's surface with a VAC device (Vacuum Assisted Closure, Advanced Therapy System).

Polyurethane (PU) or polyvinyl-alcohol (PVA) foam is cut to fit the wound cavity precisely to achieve negative pressure on the wound surface. PU foam is black and easily deformable, while PVA (white) foam is stiffer and requires higher pressures.

Most doctors use TNP therapy at 125 mm Hg (sub-atmospheric pressure) using black PU foam – which means 125 mm Hg below atmospheric pressure. Evidence that this is the optimal pressure is limited. Morykwas showed, using laser Doppler flow probes in an acute wound pig model, that local tissue perfusion increased with increasing pressure up to 125 mm Hg. Although, a further increase in pressure decreased local tissue perfusion, giving a bell-shaped distribution.

TNP dressings should be changed every 48-56 hours except in exceptional circumstances (for example, with a skin graft). Manufacturers recommend changing dressings more often in case of (aerobic) infection. If dressings are routinely left for more extended periods (more than 56 hours), this may lead to increased discomfort during dressing change due to the ingrowth of granulation tissue into the foam. Anecdotal findings are that granulation tissue is clinically less healthy the longer the dressing is left in situ, although no published literature exists on this topic.

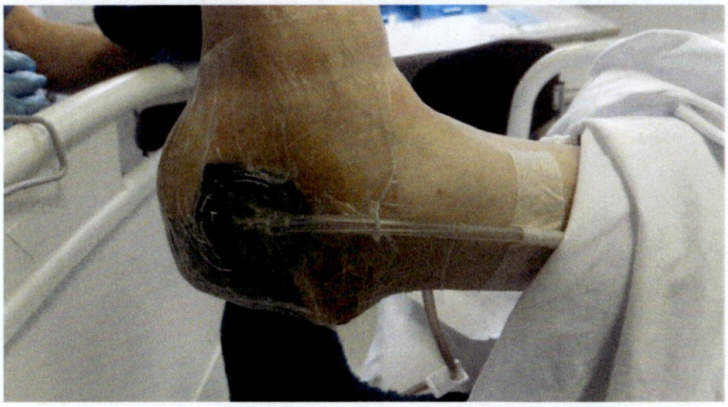

Figure 4.6 VAC system operation diagram (source: Department of Vascular Surgery VUSCH).

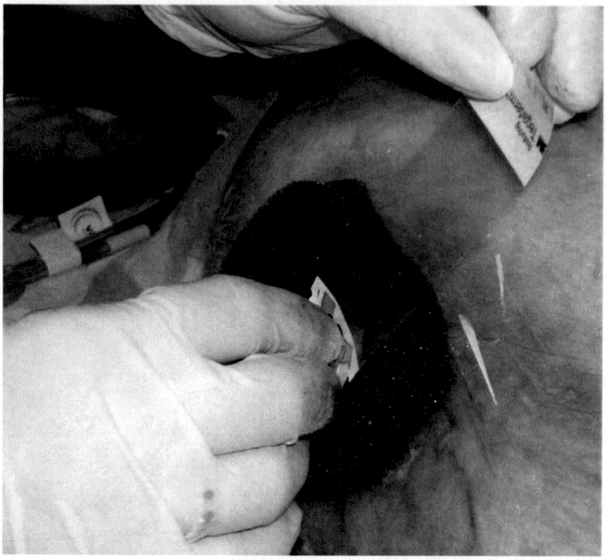

Figure 4.7 Implantation of the VAC system (source: Department of Vascular Surgery VUSCH).

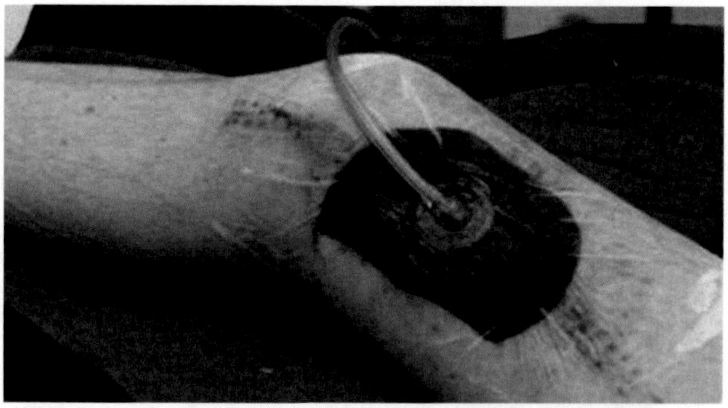

Figure 4.8 VAC system on a dehiscent wound (source: Department of Vascular Surgery VUSCH).

Further pressure increases (>200 mm Hg) have been shown to decrease blood flow.

These direct effects on the dermal vasculature are thought to be mediated by influencing vasomotor mediators. However, the indirect effects of mechanical forces acting on the extracellular matrix inevitably affect the microvasculature.

Increasing mechanical stress in vitro causes an increase in cellular activity, the nature of which varies by cell type and methodology. Accelerated cell growth and DNA synthesis were observed. Experimental evidence from model systems suggests mechanical forces can lead to increased fibrogenesis in skin wound models. The resulting reduction in edema is thought to help improve blood and nutrient flow to the wound. However, removing exudate (which will include metalloproteinases and other inflammatory mediators) from the wound and edema from the surrounding tissues promotes the movement of nutrients to the wound area, even if there is no increased blood flow. The removal of fluid prevents the accumulation of inflammatory mediators and promotes the diffusion of additional nutrients into the wound. All of these are beneficial to the healing process, especially in chronic wounds, where it is thought that an imbalance of metalloproteinases can impede recovery. Anecdotally, the volume of wound exudate obtained from acute wounds decreases significantly during the first three to four days, reducing wound edema. However, there is currently no quantitative evidence to support an actual reduction in wound interstitial fluid, although studies are ongoing to attempt to evaluate changes in wound fluid components under TNP.

Acute wounds

After the excision of any non-viable tissue, the application of TNP therapy for two to three weeks can prevent local infection, partially fill the wound with granulation tissue, and transform difficult-to-manage situations into simpler circumstances, for example, the production of exposed granulation tissue at the wound bed, which can be easily covered with a skin graft. It can stimulate the formation of granulation tissue on the bone. This is an essential advantage in elderly or debilitated patients, where the number of amputations can be reduced.

Chronic wounds are defined as not healing in the expected time. In elderly patients, nutritional deficiencies and polypathology may prevent reconstructive surgery. Surgery in patients with neurological deficits can be challenging to treat due to the absence of neurotrophic factors to protect the wound and their increased propensity for infection. The use of surgery for these wounds is thus often limited to those cases where improvement can be expected. TNP therapy can keep the wound clean while simultaneously stimulating granulation tissue, reducing the reconstruction requirements of an individual wound. The usefulness of TNP has been demonstrated in complex diabetic ulcers, chronic ulcers, and decubitus ulcers.

Protocols for TNP therapy use must be tailored to the specific treatment goals of the individual patient. Therefore, if the purpose of treatment is to fill the wound cavity with granulation tissue, then the dressing is regularly changed at two-day intervals until the cavity is reduced. However, if TNP is used to secure the skin graft, the dressing is left in place for five days at lower pressure (75 mm Hg sub-atmospheric pressure).

TNP therapy can be used to help move the reconstructive requirements of the wound down the reconstructive ladder. This can result in many potential benefits for the patient and treatment regimen. For example, a wound requiring flap reconstruction can be reduced, and a healthy wound bed can be created to enable the application of a skin graft, a simple procedure, instead of the more difficult flap reconstruction.

Manufacturers recommend that TNP dressings are routinely changed at 48-hour intervals. If the foam dressing adheres to the wound bed during a dressing change, saline or, alternatively, lidocaine may be applied to the foam to moisten the adhesion sites; between dressing changes, the treatment should be active for more than 22 hours each day. Dressings should also be removed if TNP therapy is completed, as the foam and adhesive layer are not designed to absorb exudate. This would result in a macerated and congested wound.

TNP therapy is considered most effective at a pressure of 125 mm Hg. However, clinical studies to date have not confirmed this. Treatment should be discontinued when wound goals are achieved or if infection or lack of progress is noted.

Contraindications

TNP is not successful on grossly infected wounds. The wound bed needs to be cleaned using surgical or topical exfoliating agents. TNP therapy is also not recommended for use in bleeding wounds, or malignant diseases, directly on an artery or necrotic tissue. The presence of abnormal coagulation, fistulas, open body cavities, or after oncological resections should be considered and evaluated individually. Clinical judgment of potential benefits should be used in each case.

However, reports show that increased healing time and a reduction in the number of required operations correlate with reduced overall care costs. It should also enable the treatment of larger wounds in the community with minimal impact on nursing care. This would free up hospital beds.

Comprehensive prevention and therapy of the diabetic foot can reduce the number of amputations by 50% and significantly reduce the cost of long-term treatment. In all countries, foot care management should be organized at GP, and podiatry nurse level, and specialist foot centers with diabetologists, podiatry nurses, radiologists, general, orthopedic, and vascular surgeons, orthopedic technicians, and physiotherapists should be established.

References

Argenta LC, Morykwas MJ. Vacuum-assisted closure: a new method for wound control and treatment: clinical experience. Ann Plast Surg1997;38:563–76.

Banwell PE, Jones SM, Evison D. Topical negative pressure modulates dermal microvascular blood flow dynamics and temperature profiles at the wound-dressing interface. J Wound Care. (in press).

Banwell PE, Teot L. Topical negative pressure (TNP): the evolution of novel wound therapy. J Wound Care2003;12:22–8.

Beitz JM , Bates-Jensen B. Algoritmy, kritické cesty a počítačový softvér pre starostlivosť o rany: súčasný stav a budúci potenciál. Manažment stomických rán 2001 ; 47 : 33 – 40.

Curtis AS, Seehar GM. The control of cell division by tension or diffusion. Nature1978;274:52–3.

Evans D, Land L. Topical negative pressure for treating chronic wounds. Cochrane Library. Issue 1. Oxford: Update Software, 2001.

Fabian TS, Kaufman HJ, Lett ED, et al. The evaluation of subatmospheric pressure and hyperbaric oxygen in ischemic full-thickness wound healing. Am Surg2000;66:1136–43.

Fay MF . Drenážne systémy. Ich úloha pri hojení rán. AORN J 1987 ; 46 : 442-55 .

Fleischmann W, Becker U, Bischoff M, et al. Vacuum sealing: indication, technique, and results. European Journal of Orthopaedic Surgery and Traumatology1995;5:37–40.

Fox JW , Golden GT. Použitie drénov pri podkožných chirurgických zákrokoch. Am J Surg 1976 ; 132 : 673 –4.

Garner GB, Ware DN, Cocanour CS, et al. Vacuum-assisted wound closure provides early fascial reapproximation in trauma patients with open abdomens. Am J Surg2001;182:630–8.

Giovanni UM, Demaria RG, Otman S, et al. Treatment of poststernotomy wounds with negative pressure. Plast Reconstr Surg2002;109:1747.

Greer SE, Longaker MT, Margiotta M, et al. The use of subatmospheric pressure dressing for the coverage of radial forearm free flap donor-site exposed tendon complications. Ann Plast Surg1999;43:551–4.

Gustafsson R, Johnsson P, Algotsson L, et al. Vacuum-assisted closure therapy guided by C-reactive protein level in patients with deep sternal wound infection. J Thorac Cardiovasc Surg2002;123:895–900.

http://www.nczisk.sk

Jirkovská, A.: Infekce u syndromu diabetické nohy, In: Jirkovská,. A a spol.: Syndrom diabetické nohy, Praha, Maxdorf2006; 176–199.

Joseph E, Hamori CA, Bergman S, et al. A prospective randomized trial of vacuum-assisted closure versus standard therapy of chronic nonhealing wounds. Wounds2000;3:60–7.

Levin LS . Rekonštrukčný rebrík. Ortoplastický prístup. Orthop Clin North Am 1993 ; 24 : 393-409 .

Morykwas MJ, Argenta LC, Shelton-Brown EI, et al. Vacuum-assisted closure: a new method for wound control and treatment: animal studies and basic foundation. Ann Plast Surg1997;38:553–62.

Morykwas MJ, David LR, Schneider AM, et al. Use of subatmospheric pressure to prevent progression of partial-thickness burns in a swine model. J Burn Care Rehabil1999;20:15–21.

Morykwas MJ, Faler BJ, Pearce DJ, et al. Effects of varying levels of subatmospheric pressure on the rate of granulation tissue formation in experimental wounds in swine. Ann Plast Surg2001;47:547–51.

Mullner T, Mrkonjic L, Kwasny O, et al. The use of negative pressure to promote the healing of tissue defects: a clinical trial using the vacuum sealing technique. Br J Plast Surg1997;50:194–9.

Philbeck TE Jr, Whittington KT, Millsap MH, et al. The clinical and cost-effectiveness of externally applied negative pressure wound therapy in the treatment of wounds in home healthcare Medicare patients. Ostomy Wound Manage1999;45:41–50.

Porter R. Chirurgia. Krv a črevá krátka história medicíny . Londýn: Penguin, 2002 : 109 – 34.

Rybka, Jaroslav: Diabetes mellitus – komplikace a přidružená onemocnění, Grada Publishing, a. s., 1. 1. 2007 – 317 strán, s. 238 – 253.

Schneider AM, Morykwas MJ, Argenta LC. A new and reliable method of securing skin grafts to the difficult recipient bed. Plast Reconstr Surg1998;102:1195–8.

Sibbald RG, Mahoney J. A consensus report on the use of vacuum-assisted closure in chronic, difficult-to-heal wounds. Ostomy Wound Manage2003;49:52–66.

Urschel JD, Scott PG, Williams HT. The effect of mechanical stress on soft and hard tissue repair; a review. Br J Plast Surg1988;41:182–6.

Chapter 5

Diabetic Foot and Radiological Findings

Martina Zavacká, MD*

Department of Vascular Surgery, East Slovak Institute of Cardiovascular Diseases, Faculty of Medicine, Pavol Jozef Šafárik University in Košice, Slovakia

Abstract

Early and correct diagnosis of diabetic foot syndrome affects the prognosis and reduces the risk and necessity of amputation of the affected limb. Today, the role of the diagnostic and interventional radiologist is irreplaceable. It allows not only diagnosis but also early and less invasive treatment. Conventional digital subtraction angiography (DSA), CT, or MR angiography are necessary for planning endovascular surgery and vascular surgery reconstructions.

Key Words: diagnosis, amputation, diabetic foot, digital subtraction angiography (DSA), MR angiography, CT angiography

Early and correct diagnosis of diabetic foot syndrome affects the prognosis and reduces the risk and necessity of amputation of the affected limb. Today, the role of the diagnostic and interventional radiologist is irreplaceable. It enables diagnosis and early and less invasive treatment of arterial damage caused by diabetes. The main problem is the early diagnosis of osteomyelitis. Diagnosing it early and correctly, differentiating it, and choosing the proper treatment is essential. The basis is an X-ray image, which is relatively cheap and the most accessible. It is necessary to make two projections: oblique and anteroposterior. However, it may not show osteomyelitis in the early stages. At an early stage, the sensitivity of changes in the bone skeleton is up to 60-75%, specificity

* Corresponding Author's Email: martina.zavacka@upjs.sk

In: Diabetic Foot
Editor: Martina Zavacká
ISBN: 979-8-89113-019-7

of 60-90%. However, confirming the bones' osteoarthropathy and obtaining a detailed anatomical overview of the lower limb bones, deformations, and emphysema is possible. Osteitis and osteoarthropathy gradually deform and fragment the bones; therefore, repeated X-ray images in time are necessary for patients with diabetic foot syndrome. In Möckenberg's sclerosis, X-ray examination reaches 99% sensitivity. A characteristic finding is the calcification of the dorsal artery. X-ray densitometry is also of great importance for the diagnosis of Charcot osteoarthropathy. It shows differences in bone mineralization density.

Other imaging modalities include computed tomography (CT), magnetic resonance (MR), ultrasonography, scintigraphy, or CT examination with labeled leukocytes.

Using color and Doppler imaging, we examine the arterial and venous systems of the lower limbs. We can identify the extent of stenoses and arterial occlusions or rule out venous system thrombosis. Today, the method is easily available and repeatable. However, in the case of swelling or cellulitis of the diabetic foot, imaging of the crural arteries is limited. It may help assess muscle atrophy.

Conventional digital subtraction angiography (DSA), CT angiography (CTAG), or MR angiography is necessary for planning endovascular intervention and vascular surgical reconstruction. CTAG is a non-invasive method; it also shows the arterial system from the abdominal aorta in a distal direction. The disadvantage is the asymmetric flow rate through one limb, the image quality is lower in patients with low cardiac output, and the administration of a larger amount of contrast substance, which is limiting in patients with impaired renal functions. MRA is relatively accurate in quantifying stenoses of the arterial system, but it is limited by the presence of massive calcifications and the inaccuracy in distinguishing tight stenoses from occlusions. We use it in case of allergy to contrast substance and patients with renal insufficiency. The disadvantage is the price, availability, and length of the examination.

In addition to assessing vascular structures, CT also allows the assessment of damage to bone structures, destruction of the skeleton, cortical destruction,

Table 5.1 Eichenholtz classification (Sanverdi, 2012)

stage		
0	Risk patient – diabetic neuropathy, acute injury	X-ray image: normal
I	Fragmentation – edema, erythema	X-ray image: bone fragmentation
II	Coalescence – regression of edema, erythema	X-ray image: connecting fragments
III	Consolidation - without edema and erythema	X-ray image: fracture remodeling

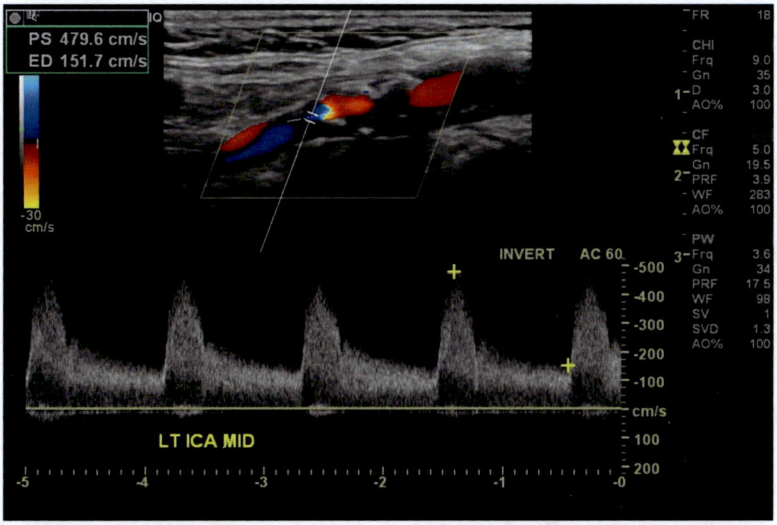

Figure 5.1 USG imaging of femoral artery stenosis (source: Department of Vascular Surgery VUSCH).

gas bubbles, sequestrations, and their relationship to the surrounding structures. Due to its high sensitivity, magnetic resonance (MR) can distinguish neuroarthropathy from inflammatory impairment of soft tissues, but not the early stages of osteomyelitis and osteoarthropathy. However, it remains the primary method in the diagnosis of Charcot osteoarthropathy. A particular disadvantage of CTAG and MRAG remains the lower quality imaging of peripheral arteries and control of the patency of the intervened sections of the peripheral arteries. MR allows us to distinguish between vital and necrotically changed tissues and bones, which is essential when planning surgical intervention. Bone marrow signal changes in osteomyelitis and the acute stage of osteoarthropathy are identical. Edema, which in osteoarthropathy has a juxta-articular localization and affects several joints in the subchondral region, can be helpful for differentiation. In osteomyelitis, only one bone is involved, and the marrow edema is more diffuse, mainly in the phalanges, metatarsal heads, and calcaneus. With a fluid collection inside the bone, we assume a bone abscess. Fractures - most often of the calcaneus - can be present with osteoporosis and neuropathic changes. With the help of MR, we can also evaluate secondary signs of infection: ulcers, fistulas, abscesses, cellulitis, and tendosynovitis.

Scintigraphy will enable the visualization of metabolic and functional tissue changes. The image is created by ionizing radiation that emanates from the patient's body. The source is a radiopharmaceutical substance distributed into the tissues using a carrier. The most frequently used is 99mTc. The advantage

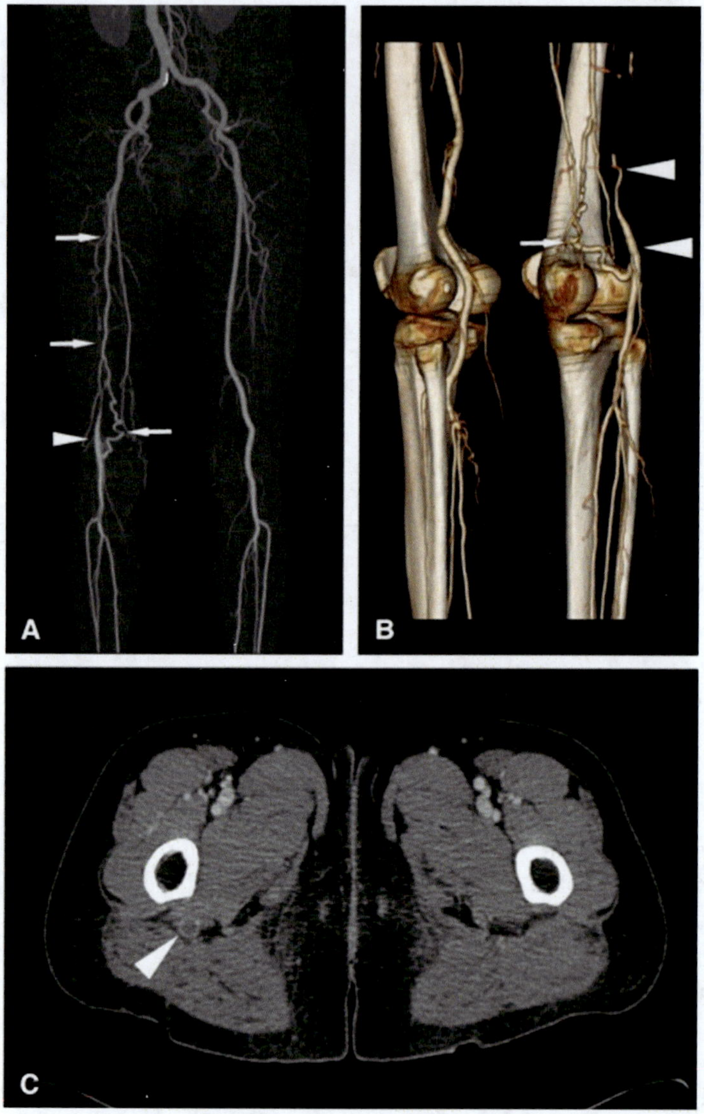

Figure 5.2 CTAG image of the arteries of the lower limbs: A) anteroposterior view, B) 3D image, C) transversal section (source: Department of Vascular Surgery VUSCH).

is a low dose of radiation; the disadvantage is a worse spatial resolution of the exact localization of the radiopharmaceutical. Skeletal scintigraphy uses pathophysiological changes that occur during inflammation. In the bone tissue, the flow, permeability of capillaries, and metabolic turnover of osteoclasts and osteoblasts increase. The method has a high sensitivity but is relatively non-specific.

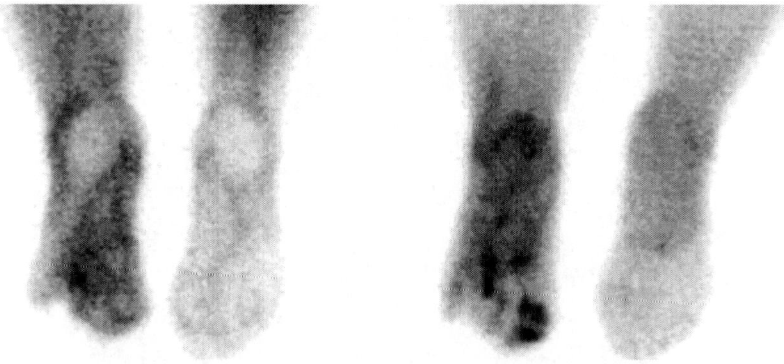

Figure 5.3 Scintigraphy of the lower limbs with labeled leukocytes (source: Department of Vascular Surgery).

It does not distinguish between infectious and non-infectious inflammation. In leukocyte-labeled scintigraphy, leukocytes are labeled with 99mTc and accumulate at the site of inflammation. However, they also accumulate in non-infectious inflammation, and their sensitivity is low in chronic inflammation. The method has meaning, e.g., when deciding on amputating (part of) a limb. Amputation is highly probable if the increased accumulation of leukocytes persists after 3-4 weeks of antibiotic therapy. Scintigraphy with polyclonal human immunoglobulin G is also commonly used. The disadvantages of scintigraphy methods are the low availability, length, and interpretation of the examination.

Despite the progress of other imaging methods, digital subtraction angiography (DSA) remains the "gold standard" in imaging methods of lower limb arteries. We perform it by retrograde puncture of the common femoral artery, introducing a diagnostic catheter into the abdominal aorta. By injecting contrast material, we gradually visualize the abdominal section of the aorta, the pelvis' arteries, and the lower limbs' arteries. This allows us to make an accurate decision about the following therapeutic process (endovascular) or to plan an angiosurgical procedure on the arteries.

Bone and joint complications of diabetic foot syndrome

Osteomyelitis

20-65% of patients with diabetic foot syndrome suffer from osteomyelitis. It is typically located in the leg's front and calcaneus areas. On the X-ray image in the early stage, we find cortical erosions, periostosis, lysis of the cortical part, pyarthrosis, edema of soft tissues, gas, or osteoporosis. However, the X-ray

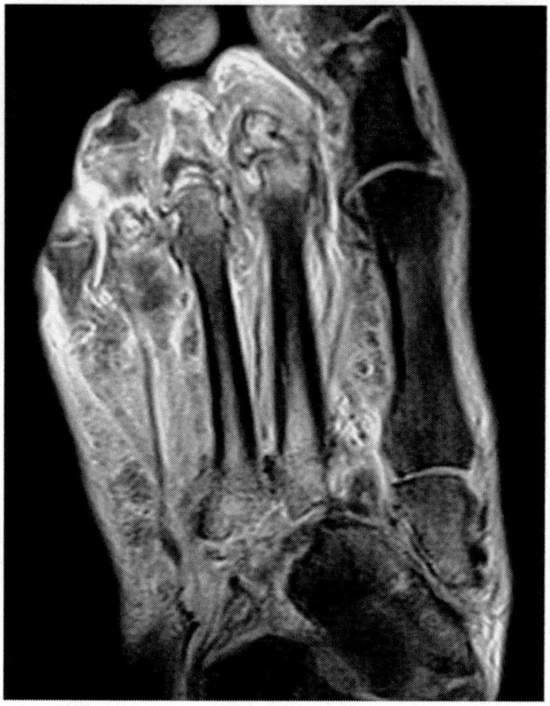

Figure 5.4 Osteomyelitis of the right foot in the MR image (source: Department of Vascular Surgery VUSCH).

findings are mostly negative in the first two weeks. It is primarily detected by an MR examination (spreading of the skin ulcer towards the bone and bone marrow), secondarily by a visible reaction of the periosteum. However, this secondary sign is better visible on the X-ray image. In chronic stages, the bone is sclerotic, mottled, loses its structure, the medullary cavity disappears, and joint ankylosis and leg deformities occur.

(Charcot's) Neuroarthropathy

It is a form of diabetic foot affecting the bones and joints. It is a relatively rare complication of peripheral diabetic neuropathy (0.8-8%) of diabetics. Neuroarthropathy of the autonomic nervous system worsens the blood supply to the joints and bones of the feet. The tarsometatarsal joints are affected, which is why the longitudinal arch of the foot collapses. Clinically, it manifests as edema, later as bone fragmentation, so the foot becomes a "skin bag" filled with bone fragments. X-ray images are negative in the early stages, and MR examination is more conclusive.

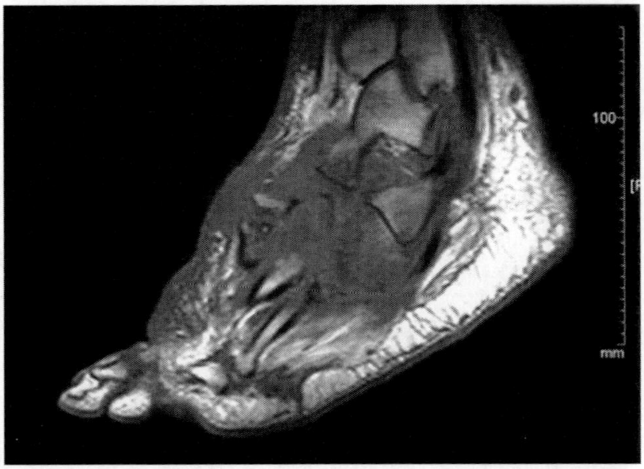

Figure 5.5 MR image of Charcot osteoarthropathy of the feet (source: Department of Vascular Surgery VUSCH).

Septic arthritis

It arises by direct hematogenous spread from the surrounding soft tissues. Affected joints are usually located near the skin ulceration (ankle, metatarsophalangeal, interphalangeal joints). The MR examination is the most helpful; it shows a complex intra-articular effusion with synovial enhancement. It may suggest neuroarthropathy of the foot.

Tendon and muscle complications in diabetic foot syndrome

Bacterial myositis and necrotizing fasciitis

It is part of an already ongoing soft tissue infection in the diabetic foot. The MR image shows edema and irregular thickening around the necrotic muscle groups. Secondarily, an intramuscular abscess and pyomyositis can occur, where the border of the deep fascia is disturbed in the MR image.

Septic tenosynovitis

It affects the peroneal tendons near the ulcer and ulcerations, most often the Achilles tendon at the calcaneus. It involves the flexor tendons on the forefoot. The MR image depicts it as a peri-tendinous enhancement of cellulite. It is

Table 5.2 Brodsky's anatomical classification in neuroarthropathy (Miller, 2006)

Type	Affected joints
1	Tarsometatarsal, navicular-cuneiform joints
2	Subtalar, talonavicular, calcaneocuboid joints
3A	Tibiotalar joint
3B	Fracture of the tuberosity of the calcaneus
4	Combination of affected areas
5	Isolated impairment of the forefoot

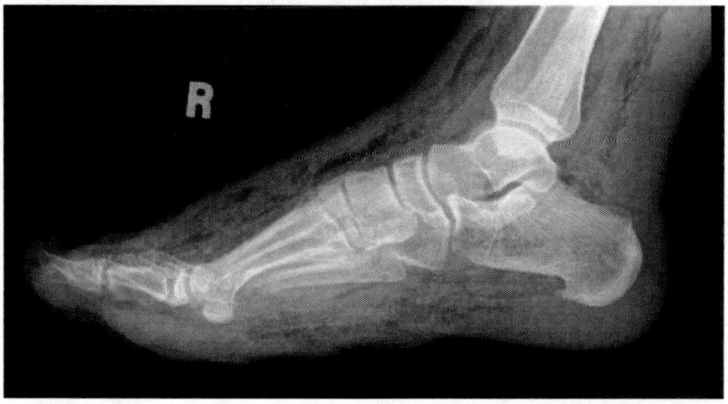

Figure 5.6 X-ray image of fasciitis of the right foot in diabetic foot syndrome (source: Department of Vascular Surgery VUSCH).

often associated with osteomyelitis and ongoing infection. The fluid in the ventral tendon capsule is non-physiological, caused by damage.

Soft tissue complications in diabetic foot syndrome

Ulcers-ulcerations

They are preceded by skin calluses, with the breakdown of the skin cover. Sensory and autonomic neuropathy, which causes skin dryness and cracking, also contributes to them. In the MR image, a breakdown of the skin line and a soft tissue defect is visible. If the size of the ulceration is more than 2 cm, the risk of developing osteomyelitis is 55-90%. With a size of more than 4.5 cm and a depth of more than 3 mm, the probability of developing osteomyelitis increases threefold.

Table 5.3 Wagner classification of ulcers (Young, 2002)

Grade 0	No ulcer/high-risk foot - deformity, calluses, Charcot's foot
Grade 1	A superficial ulcer of symmetrical thickness
Grade 2	A deeper ulcer / penetrates the tendon, not the bones/
Grade 3	A deeper ulcer with bone involvement - osteitis
Grade 4	Partial gangrene /finger, lower leg/
Grade 5	Gangrene of the entire foot

Gangrene

It is soft tissue necrosis. Clinically, we distinguish between dry and wet gangrene based on the presence/absence of infection. When wet, visible gas spreads relatively quickly, and surgical intervention is necessary. During the MR examination, devitalized soft tissue is visible, with visible edges toward healthy tissue. When necrotic tissue liquefies, a fluid signal appears. In wet gangrene, non-enhancing devitalized tissue is present, with more gas.

Cellulitis

It is an acute necrotizing inflammatory process. It affects the skin and subcutaneous tissue, not the deep structures of muscles and fascia. In the MR image, the subcutaneous tissue's normal signal density and diffuse enhancement are lost, and the edges are poorly defined. There is also an accumulation of gas in the infected part. Like MR, a CT scan can reveal skin edema and thickening of the subcutaneous tissue.

Abscess

On MR examination, it appears as a circumscribed, enlarging collection with a signal intensity typical of fluids. It is located near the entry point of infection and breakdown of the skin cover or the fascial compartments. It is easily overlooked in the case of tissue edema, so it is preferable to administer a contrast agent to visualize it. They often communicate with tendon sheaths, joints, and bony structures where they pass through. We observe them in 10-50% of patients with foot infections.

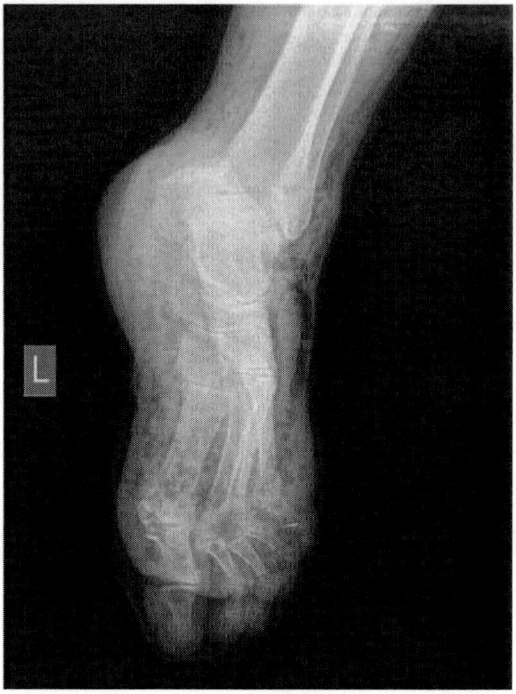

Figure 5.7 X-ray image of gangrene of the left foot (source: Department of Vascular Surgery VUSCH).

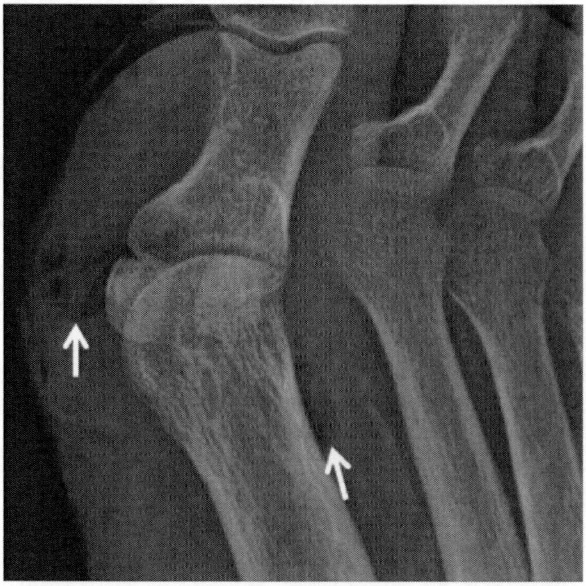

Figure 5.8 X-ray image of the abscess of the right foot (source: Department of Vascular Surgery VUSCH).

References

Lipsky, BA et al.: 2012 Infectious Diseases Society of America Clinical Practice Guideline for the Diagnosis and treatment of Diabetic Foot Infections, Clin Inf Dis 54,2012: 132-173

Low, KTA et al.: Magnetic resonance imaging of diabetic foot complications, Singapore Med J, 2015, 56(1):23-34

Miller, JC: Osteomyelitis and the diabetic foot, Radiol Rounds, 4, 2006:1-4

Peterson, N., et al.: Diagnostic Imaging of Diabetic Foot Disorders, Foot and Ankle International, 2017, Vo. 38(1) 86-95

Ranachowska, C.: et al.: Diagnostic imaging of the diabetic foot, Nuclear medicine Review, 2010, Vol.13, No.1, pp:18-22

Sanverdi, SE, et al.: Current challenges in imaging of the diabetic foot, Diabetic Foot and Ankle, 2012, 3:1, 18754

Stoller, D. et al.: Magnetic Resonance Imaging in Orthopedics and Sports Medicine, 3rd edition, Lippicont Williams and Wilkins, 2007

Young, N. et al.: Complications with outpatient angiography and interventional procedures, Cardiovasc Intervent Radiol 25,2002:123-126

Chapter 6

A Surgical Perspective on Interventional and Endovascular Procedures

Martina Zavacká, MD*
Department of Vascular Surgery, East Slovak Institute of Cardiovascular Diseases, Faculty of Medicine, Pavol Jozef Šafárik University in Košice, Slovakia

Abstract

The basis of peripheral arterial disease (PAD) is acute or chronic reduction or cessation of blood flow due to pathological changes in the arteries of the distal aorta, iliac arteries, and arteries of lower limbs. PAD of the limbs is most often caused by atherosclerosis; it reduces the quality of life and often leads to limb amputation. Since atherosclerosis is a systemic disorder, it significantly increases the risk of heart attack, stroke, and death. In 2000, the so-called Transatlantic Consensus (TASC) was established under the leadership of Prof. J.A. Dormandy and R.B. Rutherford. Endovascular treatment is chosen for morphological types A and B (according to TASC). Type C and D are more suitable for surgical treatment of peripheral arterial disease.

Key Words: peripheral arterial disease, atherosclerosis, amputation, angiosurgical reconstruction, transatlantic consensus

In 2000, the so-called Trans-Atlantic Inter-Society Consensus (TASC) was established under the leadership of Professor J.A. Dormandy and R.B. Rutherford. Sixteen European and North American professional companies participated in its processing. From the point of view of endovascular treatment, this document summarizes the clinical and morphological indications,

* Corresponding Author's Email: martina.zavacka@upjs.sk

In: Diabetic Foot
Editor: Martina Zavacká
ISBN: 979-8-89113-019-7

success, and complications of chronic and acute ischemia of the lower limbs, with a proposal for further monitoring of the success of this treatment.

The ischemic disease of the lower limbs

The basis of the disease is an acute or chronic reduction or cessation of blood flow due to pathological changes in the arteries, distal aorta, iliac arteries, and arteries of the lower limbs (Štvrtinová et al., 2006). While anatomically it is defined as an atherosclerotic disease of the arteries, functionally, it is an arterial narrowing that causes a disproportion between the supply and usage of oxygen, manifested by symptoms such as intermittent claudication, limitation of movement or tissue loss (Asahara et al., 1999).

In recent years, the name 'peripheral arterial disease' (PAD) or 'peripheral arterial occlusive disease' (PAOD) has been used for diseases of the peripheral arteries ending in ischemia.

The peripheral arterial disease also includes other arterial bloodstream diseases, except coronary arteries. PAOD of the limbs is most often caused by atherosclerosis, reduces the quality of life, and often leads to limb amputation. Because atherosclerosis is a systemic disorder, it significantly increases the risk of myocardial infarction, stroke, and death (Štvrtinová et al., 2006).

Therefore, treating this disease must be complex and long-term, focusing on optimal revascularization, improvement of ankle pressures and microcirculation, elimination of rest pain, and extension of the claudication interval (Štvrtinová et al., 2008).

Chronic / Critical Limb Ischemia (CLI)

It represents the last stage of PAOD, in which macrovascular damage reduces the distal perfusion pressure so that the microcirculation and nutrient flow to the tissues of the lower limbs is severely impaired (Becker et al., 2011). The characteristic features of the clinical presentation of CLI are described with an emphasis on objective hemodynamic confirmation of a causal relationship between PAOD and clinical findings (Becker et al., 2011). CLI is associated with a high risk of amputation, disability, and death. Currently, 20-25% of CLI patients undergo primary amputation, 50-60% undergo surgical or endovascular reconstruction, and 25% are treated with medication. Without timely and responsible diagnosis and subsequent revascularization, patients with CLI are at risk of amputation or fatal consequences (Dawson et al., 2010; Allie et al., 2009). 20-25% of patients die within one year, 25-30% undergo high limb amputation, and 20% remain in the CLI stage. 25% survive without high amputation and symptoms of CLI (Dormandy, Rutherford, 2007; Norgren et al., 2007).

According to the TASC document on managing peripheral arterial disease from 2007, the clinical definition of CLI refers to all patients with chronic ischemic pain, ulcers, and gangrene of the lower extremities attributable to objectively proven occlusive arterial disease. CLI means chronicity and must be differentiated from acute limb ischemia (TASC Recommendation No. 16) (Norgren et al., 2007).

According to the Second European Consensus from 1991, CLI in diabetics and non-diabetics is defined by the following two criteria:

- persistent ischemic rest pain, requiring regular, adequate analgesic treatment for more than two weeks with systolic ankle pressure lower than 50 mmHg and/or finger systolic pressure lower than 30 mmHg
- ulcer or gangrene on the leg or fingers with systolic ankle pressure lower than 50 mmHg or finger systolic pressure lower than 30 mmHg (TASC recommendation No. 1) (Second European Consensus, 1991)

It should be emphasized that systolic ankle pressure, expressing an absolute value like ABI, is not a highly-valuable parameter in patients with possible CLI. Instead, finger pressure measurement is recommended in all patients with possible CLI (Dattilo et al., 2011; Rooke et al., 2011).

The pressure readings are false positives if the arteries are only partially compressible. In the case of a lack of compressibility, a problem may also arise

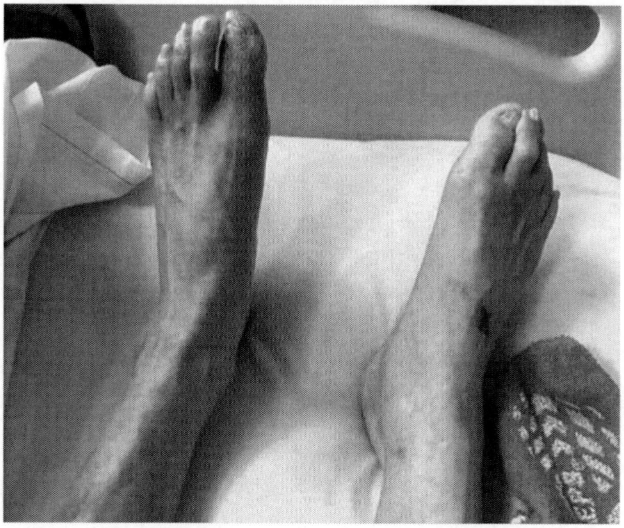

Figure 6.1 Critical limb ischemia of left lower limb (source: Department of Vascular Surgery VUSCH).

when measuring toe pressure; however, with the correct measurement of TcPO2 on the dorsum of the foot, the measured values have a high prognostic value.

Prognosis of patients with CLI

After refining the diagnosis of CLI, based on clinical and hemodynamic criteria that help to choose the proper treatment in terms of outcome and cost-effectiveness, there is a stratification of local and global risk to better identify patients from which type of treatment they could benefit the most. The BASIL study derived the predictive model designed to facilitate patient clinical decision-making. An objective measurement of the distal perfusion pressure (finger pressure) is necessary to confirm the diagnosis of CLI (de Graaff et al., 2003). Measurement of TcPO2 is probably the best non-invasive method for quantifying the degree of ischemia and assessing prognosis (Pentecost et al., 1994). Measurements on the foot's dorsum can be considered a marker of total distal outflow (run-off) and perfusion reserve. The local prognosis is good for TcPO2 values greater than 35-40 mmHg; these patients should not be classified as CLI patients. TcPO2 values of 10-35 mmHg indicate an intermediate local prognosis, and TcPO2 less than ten mmHg indicates a poor to bad prognosis (Becker et al., 2001; Johnson et al., 1988).

In a prospective study with 205 patients with CLI, defined according to the European consensus from 1991, with TcPO2 less than ten mmHg, patients were treated surgically (bypass), eventually endovascularly (PTA) with a follow-up one year after the procedure. Amputation-free survival of one year was 50%. In 75% of cases, TcPO2 values improved above 40 mmHg, and only 35% of patients had TcPO2 less than 40 mmHg (Becker et al., 2001).

Endovascular treatment is chosen for morphological types A and B (according to TASC). Type C and D are more suitable for surgical treatment of peripheral arterial disease (Štvrtinová et al., 2008).

In the last decade, there has been a reduction in surgical reconstructions and an increase in the number of PTA procedures (Al-Omran, 2003). It is advantageous for the patient if PTA immediately follows diagnostic angiography. This reduces the number of punctures and shortens the length of hospitalization. Close cooperation of the interventional radiologist/angiologist with the vascular surgeon is necessary. It is better to stop the angiography in uncertain and questionable cases and carefully consider the following therapeutic procedure.

Percutaneous transluminal angioplasty (PTA)

C. Dotter first used this method in 1966 as the so-called dotterization. He repeatedly introduced catheters with an increasing diameter into the occlusion

Table 6.1 TASC classification of femoropopliteal lesions (Štvrtinová et al., 2008)

TASC type A
1. stenosis < 3 cm
TASC type B
2. stenosis 3-10 cm long not affecting the distal course of the popliteal artery
3. severely calcified stenosis > 3 cm long
4. multiple lesions, each smaller < 3 cm /stenoses or occlusions/
5. one or multiple lesions with the absence of outflow to the foreleg arteries for enhancement inflow for distal bypass
TASC type C
6. stenosis or occlusion longer than 5 cm
7. multiple stenoses or occlusions, each 3-5 cm long or without severe calcification
TASC type D
8. complete occlusion of CFA, SFA, or complete occlusion of the popliteal artery and proximal trifurcations.

of the arteries and thus dilated them. In 1973, A.R. Gruntzig replaced this coaxial system with a balloon catheter and, in 1974, performed the first angioplasty on the femoral artery. Since then, the balloon catheter has developed considerably; mainly, its dimensions have been minimized, but the basic principle has not changed. The primary condition of successful angioplasty remains the intraluminal penetration of the conductor through the stenosis or occlusion of the artery with the introduction of a balloon catheter. Two techniques are used - retrograde (for treating ipsilateral lesions) and antegrade (puncture of the artery below the inguinal ligament). Contralateral (cross-over) approach in treating lesions on the distal and external common iliac artery and common, superficial, and deep femoral artery.

The puncture is always done in a place where compression of the artery is possible. After the wire, we introduce a sleeve with a valve, which allows us to introduce wires and catheters without significant blood loss. The coil has two lumens; one introduces the conductor, and the other serves for pressure insufflation of the balloon with a contrast agent solution and physiological solution. The balloon is insufflated at the pressure recommended by the manufacturer, generally 6-12 atm; high-pressure systems (up to 20 atm) are produced for severe stenoses. The balloon size is chosen according to the vessel size (pelvic arteries 8-10 mm, femoral 4-7 mm, popliteal arteries 4-5 mm, below the knee arteries < 4 mm).

Successful PTA is defined angiographically (as a residual stenosis of less than 15-20%), hemodynamically (no residual pressure gradient at rest or less

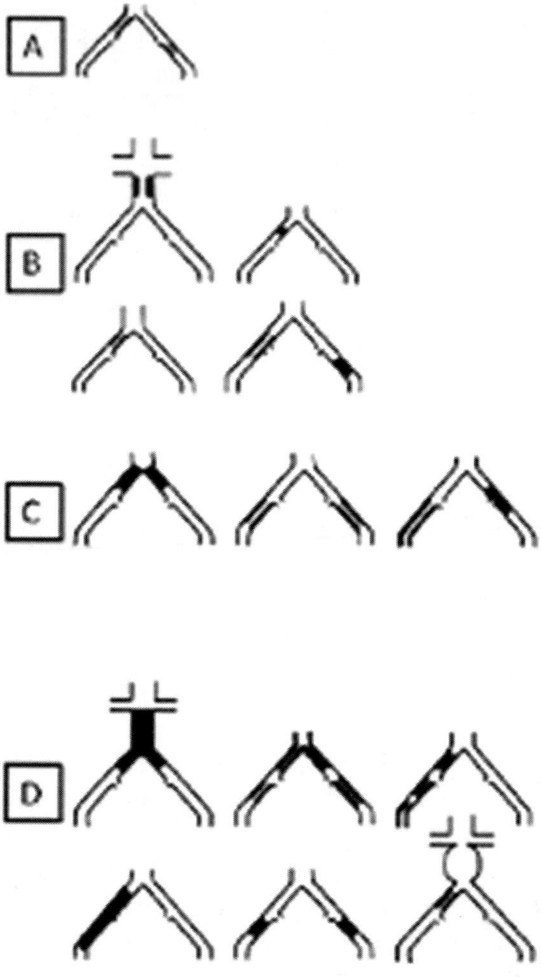

Figure 6.2 TASC classification (source: Department of Vascular Surgery VUSCH).

than 10 mm Hg after administration of nitroglycerin), or clinically (an increase in the ankle-brachial index of more than 0.15, relief of rest pains, and claudication) (Deutsch, 1941).

The most common causes of early PTA failure are early thrombosis, spasm, occlusive dissection, early elastic recoil (contraction of the blood vessel), embolization of an organized thrombus, plaque or cholesterol debris, rare vessel rupture or the formation of a pseudoaneurysm.

Restenosis due to intimal hyperplasia and chronic elastic recoil with the progression of atherosclerosis is reported as the leading cause of late PTA failure (Deutsch, 1941).

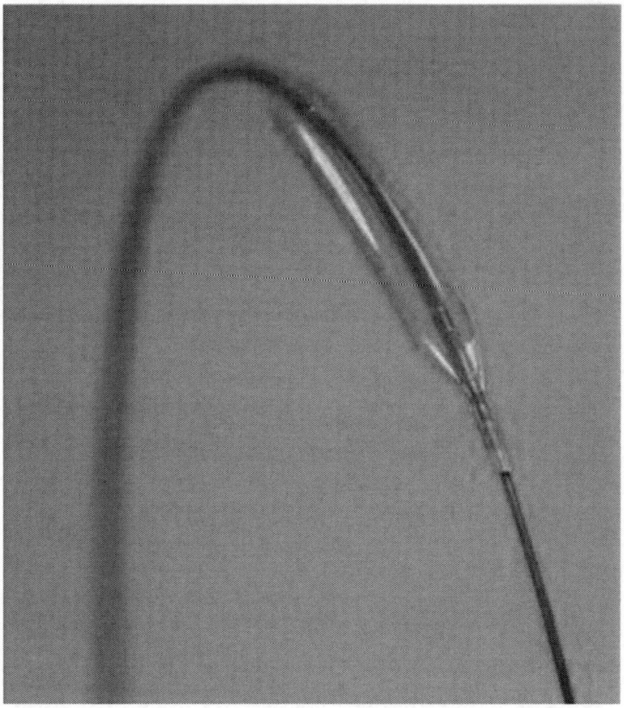

Figure 6.3 Use of a balloon in the endovascular intervention (source: Medtronic).

Stents are metal reinforcements applied to prolong the effect of PTA.

So far, we know stents: self-expandable, balloon-expandable, coated (e.g., stent-grafts), bioabsorbable, and drug-eluting stents (Štvrtinová et al., 2008). After implantation, the stent should cover the entire lesion and extend a few millimeters into the healthy vessel. We often cannot avoid overlapping collaterals, but they disappear after the original bloodstream is returned (Štvrtinová et al., 2008).

Currently, primo-implantation of the stent is recommended only to remove a complex lesion to prevent peripheral embolization. Stents significantly increase the primary success rate of PTA (up to 8-10%) because they can eliminate procedure complications (dissection, recoil). The disadvantage is their price and the occurrence of restenosis (up to 30%) inside the stent with the need for further reintervention. The classic prototype of the balloon-expandable stent is the Palmaz stent (the 1st stent approved by the FDA) for use in peripheral arteries. New generations of stents are primarily characterized by better flexibility with an effort to maintain a large radial force.

Self-expandable stents can regain their shape even after compression. They are suitable for implantation in arteries exposed to repeated pressures

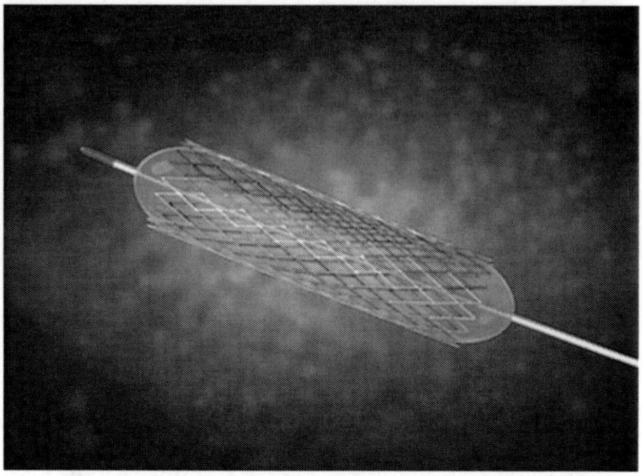

Figure 6.4 Stent with PTA balloon (source: Medtronic).

(e.g., SFA) or winding arteries (e.g., CIA). They are selected so that their diameter is 1-2 mm larger than the diameter of the blood vessel. After dilatation, the stent should not exceed the diameter of the vessel (Štvrtinová et al., 2008).

The prototype of such a stent is the wall stent, which is closed in the delivery device and, after release, expands to the original diameter in which it was made. At the same time, however, it is shortened by up to 1/3, which can cause inaccurate positioning. After implantation, the stent is dilated with a balloon catheter. Newer stents are made from nitinol, an alloy of nickel and titanium. They are more flexible than a wall stent and implant better because they shorten less. At the ends, they are equipped with contrasting marks (Štvrtinová et al., 2008).

Complications of endovascular procedures - restenosis

Restenosis can be understood as an angiographic diagnosis, defined as stenosis of 50% or more at the site of successful intervention. The location, nature, and length of the dilated artery's original involvement influence restenosis. It is necessary to distinguish between angiographic and clinical restenosis. The incidence of the clinical one is lower. More than 30% of patients with angiographic restenosis remain asymptomatic (Popma et al., 1988; Štvrtinová et al., 2008).

The discrepancy between angiographic and clinical results is probably related to the development of collateral circulation. Moderate vessel lumen loss occurs in the first 24 hours after the procedure. Stabilization or slight improvement occurs up to 1 month, and further gradual loss of vessel lumen occurs between 1 and 4 months, then a plateau phase occurs.

Recoil (early elastic narrowing), neointimal hyperplasia, and later artery remodeling are mainly involved in developing restenosis. The appearance of difficulties during the first six months after angioplasty is typical for the clinical manifestation of restenosis. A period longer than six months corresponds to further atherosclerotic damage unrelated to the angioplasty at other levels.

During 12 months, the lowest percentage of restenosis occurs in the carotid arteries (5-10%), and renal arteries (10-20%), and the most significant percentage of restenosis is present in the infrainguinal and infra-popliteal areas (30-70%) (Ahmadi et al., 2001; Rundback et al., 1998; Gray et al., 1997). Serruys (1988) reports restenosis at 1, 3, 6, and 12 months after angioplasty as 12.7%, 43%, 49%, and 52.5%, respectively.

New endovascular procedures

Subintimal (recanalization) angioplasty (SIA) is an alternative method for the impenetrability of chronic SFA occlusions. This method will cause extensive spiral dissection. A rigid catheter with slight angulation is introduced into the proximal end of the occlusion and advanced with slow pressure with minimal rotation. After the initial resistance, the catheter "jumps" a few millimeters, and its tip reaches the subintimal area. PTA / stenting can be performed after angiographic control.

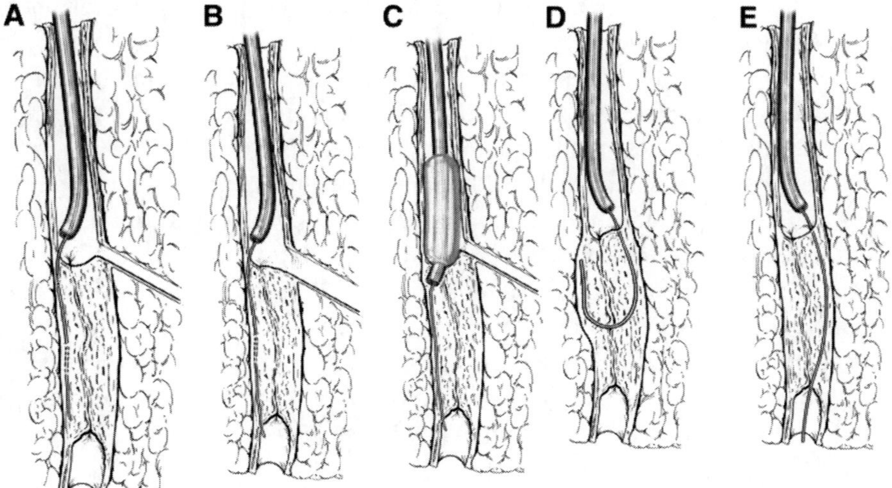

Figure 6.5 Diagram of subintimal recanalization (source: ScienceDirect.com).

The primary success rate is 76-90%, depending on the occlusion length. Complications occur in about 5% of cases. The patency rate after one year is 71%. SIA is associated with high limb salvage values within one year: 85-90%, despite low primary patency of 50%. These results were also confirmed by Bolia (2005) and Setacci (2009), with a primary success rate of 80-83.5% and a 1-year limb salvage of 85-88%.

Drug-Eluting Stents (DES)

The first substances used to cover stents were primarily intended to reduce the risk of corrosion and the negative impact of foreign material in the artery. These were, for example, chrome, titanium, platinum, ceramic materials (silicon, carbon), and polymers.

Another large group of drugs was antithrombotics (heparin, hirudin), which were supposed to reduce the risk of subacute thrombosis in the stent. However, the current combined antiplatelet treatment did not show an apparent beneficial effect of such stents covered compared to oral administration of antiplatelet drugs. No impact on late restenosis was confirmed in the studies of Karrillon et al. (1996) nor Taniuchi et al. (2001). Another attempt to reduce the incidence of restenosis, published by Van der Giessen et al. (2001), was the development of radioactive coatings with phosphorus. Unfortunately, these efforts were unsuccessful, and the use of these stents was limited.

Thus, the primary focus was developing stents as locally acting pharmaceutical carriers. The goal was to create a stable coating capable of releasing effective medications. A fundamental requirement was biocompatibility. It must not cause any adverse reaction in the vessel wall (e.g., inflammation). The drug was supposed to react with the proliferating smooth muscle cells of the media and suppress the formation of the extracellular matrix.

They were compared only with simple metallic stents in SFA in a randomized study by Duda et al. (2006) on 93 patients with claudication. Patency was assessed by ultrasound. After two years, the patencies were almost the same: 22.9% for sirolimus-coated stents vs. 21.1% for metal stents. DES stents are not yet used for femoropopliteal lesions; their role in this area is still only being investigated. DES for coronary arteries have been successfully implanted in the tibial and peroneal arteries as a revascularization treatment for CLI, but comparison with simple metallic stents is necessary (Siablis et al., 2005; Commeau et al., 2006).

Developing specialized angiological and angiosurgical departments in Slovakia improves diagnosing and treating patients with infrainguinal disabilities.

When choosing a treatment procedure for patients with severe (critical) limb ischemia (CLI), infrainguinal bypass is traditionally considered the method of choice in preventing limb amputation. Recently, however, more studies have documented the effectiveness of endovascular procedures achieving good results in saving limbs. Comparison of endovascular and surgical revascularization procedures in patients with PAOD and predominantly CLI is difficult because patient groups often differ in comorbidities, risk factors, and arterial lesions. Lesions treated with PTA are likely to be often shorter and less severe than those treated surgically. PTA is usually performed in high-risk patients with chronic renal insufficiency in the dialysis program, ischemic heart disease, heart failure, and diabetes mellitus, where surgery may be contraindicated for the clinical condition. Patients with CLI generally have a poor prognosis. However, due to the high probability of failure and the need for reintervention, PTA is recommended in patients with significant comorbidity and an expected survival of less than two years. On the other hand, infrainguinal bypass with venous graft is the method of choice for younger patients with expected more prolonged survival.

The search for the optimal method of treatment for individual patients, together with the development of surgical approaches and new endovascular techniques, leads to the need to carry out further prospective randomized clinical trials in the future to compare the long-term results of different forms of treatment considering the general condition and comorbidities of the patients.

References

ADAM, DJ et al. Bypass versus angioplasty in severe ischemia of the leg (BASIL): multicentre, randomized controlled trial. In Lancet, 2005, vol. 366, p. 1925–1934.

Ahmadi, R. et al.: Carotid artery stenting:effect of learning curve and intermediate-term morphological outcome. In JEndovasc Ther, 2001, vol. 8, p. 539-546.

ALIMI, YS et al. Efficacy of Viabahn in the treatment of severe superficial femoral artery lesions: which factors influence long-term patency? In Eur J Vasc Endovasc Surg, 2008, vol. 35, p. 346-352.

ALLIE, DE et al. 24-carat gold, 14-carat gold, or platinum standards in the treatment of critical limb ischemia: bypass surgery or endovascular intervention? In J Endovasc Ther, 2009, vol. 16, Suppl 1, p. I134-I146.

ALMAHAMEED, A. et al. Contemporary management of peripheral arterial disease: III. Endovascular and surgical management. In Cleveland Clinic Journal of Medicine, 2006, vol. 73, Suppl., p. S45-S51.

AL-OMRAN, M. Use of interventional procedures for peripheral arterial occlusive disease in Ontario between 1991 and 1998: A population-based study. In Journal of Vascular Surgery, 2003, vol 38, p. 289–295.

Asahara, T. et al.: VEGF contributes topostnatal neovascularization by mobilizing bone marrow-derived endothelialprogenitor cells. In Embo J, 1999, vol. 18, p. 3964-3972.

ATAR, E. et al. Balloon angioplasty of popliteal and crural arteries in the elderly with critical chronic limb ischemia. In Eur J Radiol, 2005, vol. 53, p. 287-92.

BAUERMEISTER, G. Endovascular stent-grafting in the treatment of superficial femoral artery occlusive disease. In J Endovasc Ther, 2001, vol.8, p. 315–320.

Becker, H. et al.: Management of Critical Limb Ischaemia and Diabetoc Foot. In Eur J Vasc Endovasc Surg, 2011, vol. 42, no. 2, p. S4-S12.

Bolia A.: Subintimal angioplasty in lower limbischemia. In J Cardiovasc Surg (Torino), 2005, vol. 46, p. 385-394.

Commeau, P. et al.: Sirolimis for below thekneee lesions: mid-term results of SiroBTK study. In Catheter CardiovascInterv, 2006, vol. 68, p. 793-798.

ČESKA, R. et al. Internal. In Triton, 2010 13. DAWSON, DL et al. Understanding objective performance goals for critical limb ischemia trials. In Semin Vasc Surg, 2010, vol. 23, no. 3, p. 129-137.

CONTE, MS Results of PREVENT III: a multicenter, randomized trial of edifoligide for the prevention of vein graft failure in lower extremity bypass surgery. In J Vasc Surg, 2006, vol. 43, p. 742-751.

Dattilo, P.B. et al.: Critical limb ischemia:endovascular strategies for limg salvage. In Prog Cardiovasc Dis, 2011, vol. 54,p. 47-60.

Dawson, D.L. et al.: Understanding objectiveperformance goals for critical limb ischemia trials. In Semin Vasc Surg, 2010, vol. 23, no.3, p. 129-137.

De Graaf, J. C. et al.: Evaluation of thepressure ant transcutaneous oxygen measurements in management of chroniccritical leg ischemia: a diagnostic rendomized clinical trial. In J VascSurg, 2003, vol. 38, p. 528-534.

Deutsch, F.: Capillary studies in raynaudsdisease. In J Lab Clin Med, 1941, vol. 26, p. 1729-1750.

Diehm, J. et al. Management of Critical Limb Ischemia and Diabetic Foot. In Eur J Vasc Endovasc Surg, 2011, vol. 42, Suppl. 2, p. S34-S39.

Dormandy J.A, Rutherford R.B.: Management of peripheral arterial disease(PAD). TASC Working Group. Transatlantic Inter-Society Consensus (TASC), J VascSurg, 2000 Jan;31(1 Pt 2): S1-S296.

Duda, S. H. et al.: Drug-eluting and barenitinol stents for the treatement of atherosclerotic lesions in the superficialfemoral artery: long-term results from the SIROCCO trial, In J Endovasc Ther, 2006,vol. 13, p. 701-710.

FARRAJ, N. et al. One-year outcomes for recanalization of long superficial femoral artery chronic total occlusions with the Viabahn stent graft. In J Invasive Cardiol, 2009, vol. 21, p. 278–281.

FEINGLASS, J. et al. Postoperative and late survival outcomes after major amputation: findings from the Department of Veterans Affairs National Surgical Quality Improvement Program. In Surgery, 2001, vol. 130, p. 21–29.

FIRT, P. et al. Vascular surgery. In Karolinum, 2006.

FRANKOVIČOVÁ, M. et al.: Vascular complications during leg reconstructive surgery, In Rozhledy v chirurgii, 1992, vol. 5, p. 251 – 253.

Gray, B.H. et al.: Limitations of PTA withstenting for femoropopliteal arterial occlusive disease. In Semin Vasc Surg,1997, vol. 10, p. 8-16.

HARTUNG, O. et al. Efficacy of Hemobahn in the treatment of superficial femoral artery lesions in patients with acute or critical ischemia: a comparative study with claudication. In Eur J Vasc Endovasc Surg, 2005, vol. 3, p. 300-306.

HENRY, M. et al. Clinical experience with the OptiMed sinus stent in the peripheral arteries. In J Endovasc Ther, 2003, vol. 10, p. 772-779.

HIRSCH, AT et al. ACC/AHA 2005 practice guidelines for the management of patients with peripheral arterial disease (lower extremity, renal, mesenteric and abdominal aortic): a collaborative report from the American Association for Vascular Surgery/Society for Vascular Surgery, Society for Cardiovascular Angiography and Interventions, Society for Interventional Radiology, Society for Vascular Medicine and Biology, and the American College of Cardiology/ American Heart Association Task Force on Practice Guidelines

Johnson, W.C. et al.: Supplemental oxygen anddependent positioning as adjunctive measures to improe forefoot tissueoxygenation. In Arch Surg, 1988, vol. 123, p. 1227-1230.

Karrillon, G. J. et al.: Intracoronary stentimplantation without ultrasound guidance and with replacement of conventionalanticoagulation by antiplatelet therapy. 30-day clinical outcome of the FrenchMulticenter Registry. In Circulation, 1996, vol. 94, p. 1519-1527.

KAWAMURA, Y. et al. Nitinol stenting improves primary patency of the superficial femoral artery after percutaneous transluminal angioplasty in hemodialysis patients: a propensity-matched analysis. In J Vasc Surg, 2009, vol. 50, p. 1057–1062.

KEDORA, J. et al. Randomized comparison of percutaneous Viabahn stent grafts vs. prosthetic femoral-popliteal bypass in the treatment of superficial femoral arterial occlusive disease. In J Vasc Surg, 2007, vol. 45, p. 10–16.

KLINKERT, P. et al. Saphenous vein versus PTFE for above-knee femoropopliteal bypass. A review of the literature. In Eur J Vasc Endovasc Surg, 2004, vol. 27, p. 357–362.

KRAJÍČEK, M. et al. Surgical and interventional treatment of vascular diseases. In Grada, 2007

KULLO, IJ et al. Ethnic differences in peripheral arterial disease in the NHLBI Genetic Epidemiology Network of Arteriopathy (GENOA) study. In Vasc Med, 2003, vol. 8, no. 4, p. 237-242.

LAIRD, JR et al. Nitinol stent implantation versus balloon angioplasty for lesions in the superficial femoral artery and proximal popliteal artery: twelve-month results from the RESILIENT randomized trial. In Circ Cardiovasc Interv, 2010, vol. 3, p. 267-276.

LAMMER, J. Femoropopliteal artery obstruction: from the balloon to the graft. In Cardiovasc Intervent Radiol, 2001, vol. 24, p. 73-83.

Norgren L. et al.: Inter-Society Consensus forthe Management of Peripheral Arterial Disease (TASC II), In Eur J Vasc EndovascSurg, 2007, vol. 33, Suppl 1, p. S1-S75.

Pentecost, M.J. et al.: Guidlines for peripheralpercutaneous transluminal angioplasty of the abdominal aorta and lowerextremity vessels. A statement for health professionals froma special writing group of the Councils on Cardiovascular Radiology,Arteriosclerosis, Cardi.Thoracic and Vascular Surgery, Clinical

Cardiology andEpidemiology and Prevention, the American Heart Associotion. In Circulation, 1994,vol. 89, p. 511-531.

Popma J.J. et al.:Long-term outcome of patients with asymptomatic restenosis after percutaneoustransluminal coronary angioplasty. In Amer J Cardiol., 1988, vol. 62, p. 1298.

Rooke, T.W. et al: 2011 ACCF/AHA FocusedUpdate of the Guidline for the Management of Patients with Peripheral ArteryDisease (Updating the 2005 Guidline): A Report of the American College ofCardiology Foundation/American Heart Association Task Force on PracticeGuidlines. In Circulation, 2011, vol. 124, p. 2020-2045.

Rundback J.H. et al.: Renal artery stentplacement for the management of ischemic nephropathy. In J Vasc Interv Radiol.,1998, vol. 9, p.413-420.

Second European consensus document on chroniccritical leg ischemia. In Circulation, 1991, vol. 84, p.IV1-IV26.

Serruys P.W. et al.: Incidence of restenosisafter succesfull coronary angioplasty: A time-related phenomen.A quantitave angiographic study in 342 consecutive patients at 1, 2, 3 and4 months. In Circulation, 1988, vol. 77,p.361.

Setacci, C. et al.: Subintimal angioplastywith the aid of a re-entry device for TASC C and D lesions of the SFA. InEur J Vasc Endovasc Surg, 2009, vol. 38, p. 76-87.

Siablis, D. et al.: Sirolimus-eluting versus bare stents for bailout aftre suboptimal infrapopliteal angioplasty for critical limb ischemia: 6-months angiographic results from a randomized prospective single-center study. In J Endovac Ther, 2005, vol. 12, no.6, p. 685-695.

Štvrtinová, V. et al.: Odporúčania pre diagnostiku a liečbu periférneho artériového ochorenia končatín. In Cardiol, 2006, vol. 15, no. 6, p. 317-323.

Taniuchi, M. et al.: Randomized comparision ofticlopidine and clopidogrel after intracoronary stent implantation ina broad patient population. In Circulation, 2001, vol. 104, p. 539-543.

Van der Giessen, W.J. et al.: Edge effect of32p radioactive stents is caused by the combination of chronic stent injury andradioactive dose fall off. In Circulation, 2001, vol. 104, p. 2236-2241.

Writing Committee to develop guidelines for the management of patients with peripheral arterial disease. In Circulation, 2005, vol. 113, no. 11, p. 463-654.

Chapter 7

Revascularization of Lower Limb Arteries and Principles of Surgical Treatment in Patients with Diabetes Mellitus

Martina Zavacká, MD*

Department of Vascular Surgery, East Slovak Institute of Cardiovascular Diseases, Faculty of Medicine, Pavol Jozef Šafárik University in Košice, Slovakia

Abstract

The goal of surgical treatment for diabetic foot syndrome is to relieve rest pain and heal defects. Bypass surgery remains the gold standard in treating long lesions of the superficial femoral artery (SFA). The great saphenous vein (GSV) is the best graft for infrainguinal bypasses. The surgery is a life-saving action for the limb. When indicated, we must also consider the nature of the underlying disease. Primary amputation without an attempt for vascular reconstruction is indicated only in the case of extensive and irreversible ischemic changes and septic gangrene.

Key Words: angiosurgical revascularization, bypass, critical limb ischemia, rest pain, ulcer

Infrainguinal reconstructions and principles of surgical treatment of diabetic foot syndrome

The goal of surgical treatment for diabetic foot syndrome is to relieve rest pain and heal defects. An ischemic defect is considered a skin integrity disorder that

* Corresponding Author's Email: martina.zavacka@upjs.sk

In: Diabetic Foot
Editor: Martina Zavacká
ISBN: 979-8-89113-019-7

does not heal due to ischemia, not just one that arose due to ischemia. (Principles of Surgery). According to the 2007 TASC document on the management of peripheral arterial disease, the clinical definition of CLI refers to all patients with chronic ischemic pain, ulcers, and gangrene of the lower limbs due to objectively proven occlusive arterial disease. CLI stands for chronicity and must be differentiated from acute limb ischemia (TASC Recommendation No. 16).

According to the Second European Consensus from 1991, CLI in diabetics and non-diabetics is defined by the following two criteria:

- persistent ischemic rest pain, requiring regular, adequate analgesic treatment for more than two weeks with systolic ankle pressure lower than 50 mmHg and/or toe systolic pressure lower than 30 mmHg
- ulcer or gangrene on the leg or toes with systolic ankle pressure lower than 50 mmHg or toe systolic pressure lower than 30 mmHg (TASC recommendation No. 1) (Second European Consensus, 1991)

It should be emphasized that systolic ankle pressure, expressing an absolute value like ABI, is not a highly-valuable parameter in patients with possible CLI. Instead, the toe pressure measurement is recommended in all patients with possible CLI.

Bypass surgery remains the gold standard in treating long lesions of the superficial femoral artery (SFA). The great saphenous vein (GSV) remains the best graft for infrainguinal bypasses. The use of an autologous vein is still preferred over a prosthesis or endovascular intervention, as it is the most flexible and durable method of revascularizing the lower limbs and saving the limb. Proximal bypasses (above the knee) using GSV have a 5-year patency rate of 77.2% in claudication patients and 69.4% in CLI patients. Distal bypasses (below the knee) sutured with GSV have similar patency (Pereira et al., 2006). Two years after the GSV graft, salvage of the limb proximally above the knee in patients with CLI is 86.9%.

Absolute indications for bypass surgery are:

- rest pain (stage III)
- (pre)gangrene of toes and/or feet (stage IV)
- good femoral inflow
- adequate popliteal run-off (however, in stages III and IV, when the progression of the disease is rapid, bypass is also indicated in patients who have only one artery of the foreleg)

Relative indications for bypass operations are:

- intermittent claudication (it is necessary to consider the ratio of risk and benefit of an operative solution when conservative therapy is not exhausted)

- young, healthy, active individuals with unilateral isolated involvement, free popliteal segment, and suitable GSV are clear candidates for classic femoropopliteal bypass

Other possible indications for bypass surgery are:

- injury causing limb ischemia
- trauma/damage to the superficial femoral artery
- cystic degeneration, popliteal artery aneurysms

The operation is a limb-saving activity. Contraindications, apart from the general risks associated with anesthesia and prolonged procedure, are almost nonexistent. The fact that limb amputation is associated with up to 60% mortality in elderly patients also contributes to this.

When indicating, we must also consider the nature of the underlying disease. While 90% of patients in atherosclerotic etiology can achieve a fundamental improvement or save the limb by revascularization, the results in inflammatory etiology are much worse. For patients with superficial femoral

Table 7.1 Indications of reconstructive arterial operations on the lower limbs (Štvrtinová et al., 2008)

I. CLINICAL INDICATION	
Clinical stage I (Fontaine)	surgery is NOT INDICATED
Clinical stage II (Fontaine)	surgery IS RELATIVELY INDICATED
Clinical stage III (Fontain)	surgery IS ABSOLUTELY INDICATED
Clinical stage IV (Fontain)	surgery IS ABSOLUTELY INDICATED
II. ANGIOGRAPHIC INDICATION	
We evaluate these criteria: 1. location and extent of occlusion, 2. quality of inflow and outflow segment ("run-in" and "run-off"), 3. caliber of vessels.	
III. GENERAL OPERATION	
We pay attention to the following: 1. severe CAD, CNS impairment, renal or respiratory insufficiency, diabetes mellitus, severe hyperlipoproteinemia, and metabolic syndrome. 2. "life expectancy" of at least two years in case of serious diseases /malignancy/ 3. morbid obesity 4. generalized impairment of the patient by an atherosclerotic process (CAD, cerebrovascular insufficiency, generalized dilatation type of atherosclerosis • anatomical reconstructions: aortoiliac endarterectomy, aorto-bifemoral bypass, iliofemoral bypass, pelvic artery endarterectomy • extraanatomical reconstructions: femoro-femoral bypass	

artery occlusion, reconstruction of only the given section is enough to improve their condition.

Primary amputation without an attempt for vascular reconstruction is only indicated for extensive and irreversible ischemic changes and septic gangrene.

The great saphenous vein (GSV) is suitable for reconstruction on the ipsilateral side in 55% of planned operations. Cumulative 2-year patency with reverse GSV is 60-70% for reconstruction below the knee cleft and 80% for bypasses above the knee cleft. 10-year secondary patency in distal FP bypasses is about 70%. Barral presented the concept of the bypass on perigenicular arteries or blind segment of the popliteal artery (assuming good perigenicular collateral circulation) in CLI patients with non-graft ratios on the popliteal artery. The 1-year primary patency in 20 patients was 85%, and limb salvage was 90%.

With venous femoropopliteal (FP) bypasses, the long-term patency and survival of the limb are significantly higher. Idu considers a vein diameter below 3.5 mm the most critical predictor of stenosis or obliteration of the venous bypass. He thinks using a composite bypass or a vein from the upper limb is better than using a small-caliber GSV. GSV harvesting can also be performed endoscopically, with fewer early complications and a better cosmetic effect. The disadvantage is the financial aspect and that the process is time-consuming.

In some cases, the non-reversed GSV sample harvesting technique is an equivalent alternative and the method of the first choice. This way, congruence between the diameter of the bypass and the recipient's vessel is achieved.

With the in situ technique, American studies with a 20-year follow-up report a 1-year cumulative patency of 91%, 5-year 81%, and 10-year 70%. In a 10-year follow-up, they observed 90% limb salvage.

Vascular prostheses from e-PTFE

According to the literature data, we expect a cumulative 5-year patency of proximal FP bypasses of 50-60%. In a series of 322 PTFE reconstructions, FP bypasses indicated for severe claudication had a primary patency of 63%, and in the case of indication for CLI, only 38%. 2/3 of all occlusions occurred within one year after surgery. Patterson reports 1-year patency of proximal FP bypass at 75%, after five years at 54%, and limb salvage at 88% and 70%, respectively. The UK Joint Vascular Research Group showed that the venoplasty interposition in the anastomotic area of proximal FP bypasses does not improve long-term patency, but plasty in the distal anastomosis site of FP PTFE bypass below the knee cleft statistically significantly improves long-term patency (52% vs. 29%). A Dutch study from 2000 reports a statistically significant difference between venous and PTFE proximal bypass patency. Two-year secondary patency of 83% in venous and 77% in PTFE bypass. Based on a 5-year follow-up, Timarana concluded that all women who used hormonal preparations are at a higher risk of occlusion of the FP bypass; with prosthetics, the risk is significantly higher. Five-year patency in female patients without hormonal treatment was 62%, and in the second group, only 22%.

Further improvement of PTFE grafts can be expected with the clinical use of in vitro endothelialized PTFE grafts using autologous endothelial cells (bone marrow, omentum). According to preliminary results, they improve the retention of endothelial cells on the surface of the graft and have a higher angiogenic potential, which helps the penetration of capillaries through the prosthesis wall. Another option is to impregnate the inner surface of the prosthesis with carbon, to which biologically active heparin (silyl-heparin) is bound, thereby increasing thromboresistance.

The long-term patency of proximal PTFE and Dacron bypasses is comparable. Green claims that the long-term patency of FP bypasses above the knee is influenced by the patient's age and the prosthesis diameter, not the material. He observed worse patency in patients younger than 65 years (men) and those with a graft diameter of less than 7 mm (regardless of the type of prosthesis).

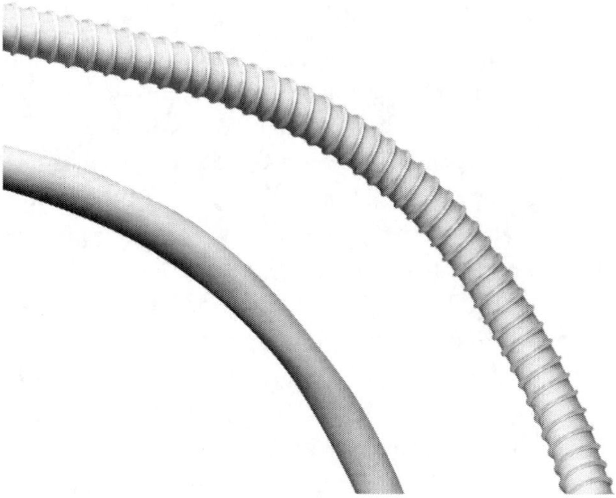

Figure 7.1 PTFE grafts (unreinforced, reinforced) (source: Department of Vascular Surgery VUSCH).

Operative procedure

Proximal and distal femoropopliteal bypass

The patient lies in a supine position, and the operated limb is rotated outwards and bent at the knee joint with support. Any trophic defects are covered before disinfecting the surgical field.

In the first step, we prepare and revise the popliteal artery through an incision on the inner side of the thigh along the front edge of the sartorius muscle in the medial femoral sulcus femoris up to the medial condyle of the femur. During dissection, we protect the GSV, which runs medially and dorsally in the subcutaneous tissue. We continue with an incision of the deep fascia of the calf, which we extend up and down. The sartorius muscle is pulled medially and dorsally. The artery is found under the tendon of the adductor magnus muscle (if necessary, we can cut it). We try to save the descending genicular artery. We remove the artery from fatty tissue and from the common sheath, where it runs with the accompanying vein. It lies medial to the artery; the nerve passes behind them. The most common site of distal anastomosis is part of the artery from the knee joint to the trifurcation. We secure the dissected artery in a sufficiently long section, 4-5 cm, with underwired tubes. We decide on a definitive reconstruction if there are no significant sclerotic changes.

Due to better results, some surgeons prefer a short (proximal) bypass, ending above the knee on the proximal segment of the popliteal artery if it is passable and has a sufficient lumen. Afterward, we dissect the common femoral artery and its branches in the groin. It is exposed from the inguinal ligament to the division into a superficial and a deep branch. Subsequently, if both dissected arteries are suitable for reconstruction, we prepare GSV from separate incisions on the thigh. We preferably use a vein from the unilateral limb. It is located more superficially in the area above the knee. Blind tunneling can damage the vein. It is necessary to estimate the length of the used vein correctly. After loosening and lifting the vein from its bed, both ends are ligated and separated. The cannula is inserted into the distal end of the vein and flushed with blood (20 ml in a 1:400,000 heparin dilution) (Frankovičová et al., 1995).

The vein is ready when sufficiently distended, its water tightness is checked, and the adventitia stripes are interrupted, making sufficient dilation possible. If the vein does not have a sufficient diameter (at least 4 mm), or if it is post-phlebitically or varicosely altered and we cannot find a vein even on the other limb, we can use a prosthesis with a diameter of 6-8 mm. The results are only slightly worse with a good outflow tract when the prosthesis is used (70% of passable grafts versus 60% of passable artificial vascular prostheses at a three-year follow-up). The tunnel for placing the bypass can

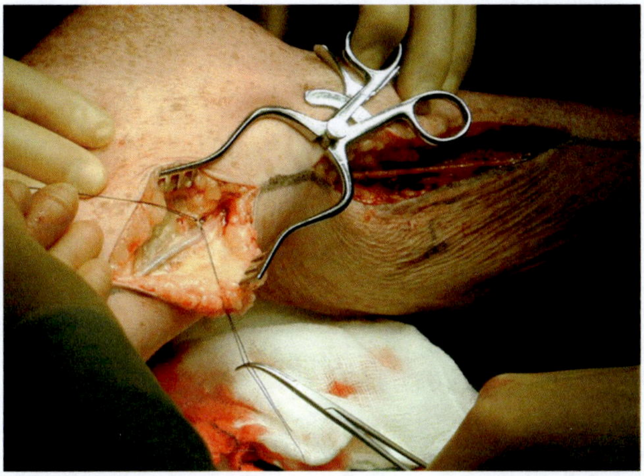

Figure 7.2 Femoropopliteal distal bypass (source: Department of Vascular Surgery VUSCH).

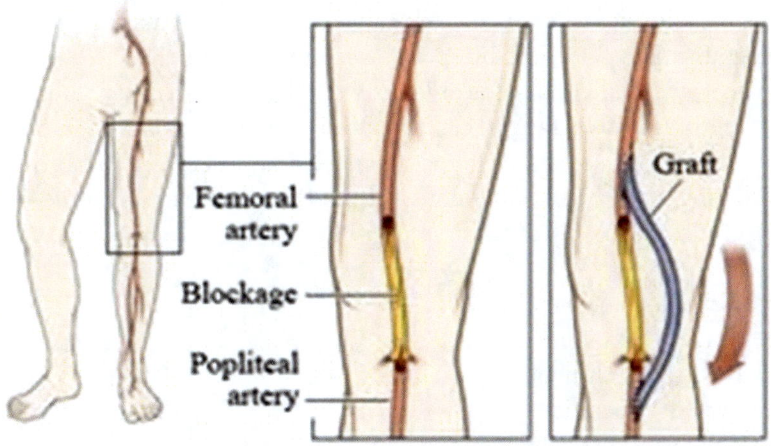

Figure 7.3 Diagram of femoropopliteal proximal and distal bypass reconstruction (source: Department of Vascular Surgery VUSCH).

be guided subcutaneously (the disadvantage is the possibility of kinking) or subfascially (it passes along Hunter's canal, under the sartorius muscle, and in front of the superficial femoral artery). The proximal end of the vein should lie above the common femoral artery and the distal end above the dissected segment without tension. After the application of 5000 IU of heparin and the application of transverse clamps, we perform an arteriotomy on the popliteal artery. The end of the GSV is cut to the length of the arteriotomy.

At this stage, by fully extending the limb, we measure the correct graft size and suture the proximal anastomosis end to side. Similarly, we suture the proximal anastomosis on the femoral artery. Just before the proximal anastomosis is finished, the proximal and distal clamps are released for a while to flush out the resulting thrombi.

Femorocrural (FC) bypass

Infrapopliteal (infragenicular)

Distal- Femoro-Tibial/Femoro-Fibular

The absolute indication for suturing the FC bypass is rest pain or an ischemic, trophic defect of the foreleg.

A crural bypass is a reconstruction in which at least one distal anastomosis is located on the trunk arteries of the lower leg (anterior tibial artery, posterior tibial artery, fibular artery, tibiofibular trunk). An autologous vein is considered the most suitable component.

Composite bypass is made from at least two types of material (vein-PTFE, autologous-allogeneic vein, bio-prosthesis-autologous vein).

The sequential bypass has at least two distal outflow anastomoses.

According to Neufang et al., the latest configurations of composite and, at the same time, sequential bypass can be composed of a bio-prosthesis in the proximal part, of an autologous vein in the distal part, with the following configuration of the distal anastomosis:

A, serial anastomosis
B, "bridge" technique
C, jump graft technique
D, inverted Y technique
E, secondary "bridge" technique

An autologous vein (GSV) can be sutured in different ways:

A, reversed
B, non-reversed
C, "IN SITU" technique (after dissecting the donor artery and the recipient crural artery, a crossectomy is performed, the proximal anastomosis is sutured with the end to the side between the CFA and the GSV, a valvulotome is introduced from its distal end towards the proximal, the venous valves are destroyed. and the distal anastomosis is sutured, stronger

inflows are eventually canceled. The advantages are that it is less time-consuming, has a better cosmetic effect, and has a preserved vein and artery congruence; the disadvantage is higher cost, leaving a larger open GSV inflow can lead to cardiac overload, and skin necrosis on the limb can occur).

D, sequential (reversing/non-reversing vein has at least two distal anastomoses, one sutured end-to-side and the other side-to-side, to ensure revascularization of multiple segments with one bypass and reduce peripheral resistance)

Suppose it is not possible to obtain a suitable GSV. In that case, the use of a prosthesis is indicated, most often PTFE in the "roof" (longitudinal extensibility), "thin wall", and "externally supported" (external reinforcement) modification. Although the technologically improved change increased the passability of bypasses, it never reached the quality of GSV.

During the implantation of prosthetic replacements, the following types of adjuvant procedures are used in the area of distal anastomosis to improve long-term patency:

1, **Interposition of an autologous venous segment**

The goal is to evenly distribute the kinetic energy of the pulse wave from the relatively rigid prosthesis to the relatively elastic artery. According to Wijesinghe's latest work, venoplasty of the distal anastomosis does not reduce the risk of myointimal proliferation. The better patency of bypasses with distal anastomosis venoplasty is explained by the fact that the anastomosis with a larger volume can accommodate the development of myointimal hyperplasia, and the stenosis of the anastomosis occurs later. The displacement and movement of the turbulence that arises in the area of the plasticized anastomosis, and thus the recipient artery in the outflow area, is often preserved (even after the bypass is closed), which allows secondary reconstructions to be carried out in the given area.

We distinguish:

1, vein cuffs (Miller's cuff, St. Mary's boot, Karacagil)
2, vein patch plasty (Taylor's, Linton's)
3, the interposition of a short venous segment (according to Jausseran)

2, **Distal anastomosis plasty using PTFE**

(Ruckert's femorocrural patch prosthesis), which minimizes the proliferative response of the arterial wall. The author confirmed it through in vitro experiments, but it did not find a wider application.

3, **AV fistula in the area of the distal anastomosis**

The goal was to reduce peripheral resistance and improve long-term patency, but it did not bring the desired effect, and this method is not recommended.

4, **Composite bypasses**

The principle is that prosthetic material is used in the femoral area (PTFE up to the height of the I., II. segment of the popliteal artery), and an autologous vein graft is used in the crural area.

We distinguish:

1, direct composite bypass
2, Hitch-Hike bypass
3, Jump bypass

According to Whittemore, the location of the distal anastomosis does not affect the long-term patency of FC bypasses but rather the healing of trophic defects. The fibular artery is considered an equivalent artery, even though it does not have its direct termination on the leg. Pedal arch patency is regarded as a reliable positive predictor of long-term bypass patency.

The optimal conditions for suturing FC bypass are:

1, the presence of a suitable autologous vein
2, patency of the pedal arch
3, at least one passing crural artery in its entire course

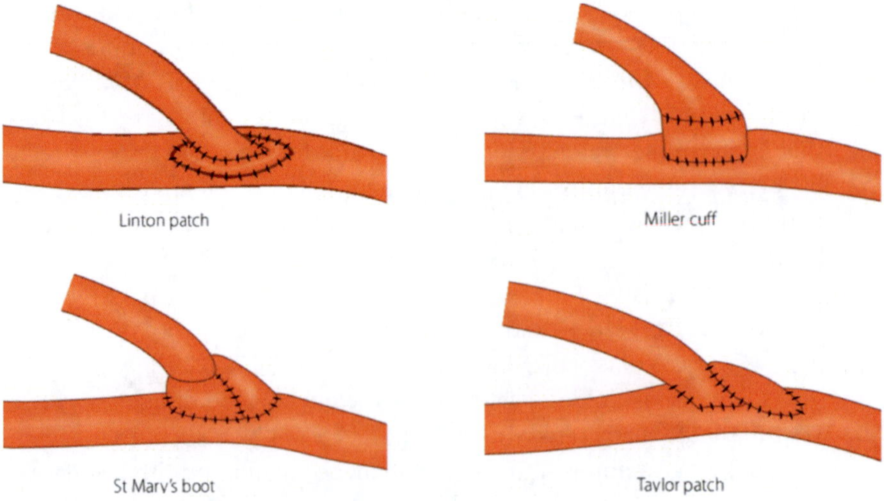

Figure 7.4 Linton's patch, St. Mary's boot, Taylor patch, and Miller cuff (source: Department of Vascular Surgery VUSCH).

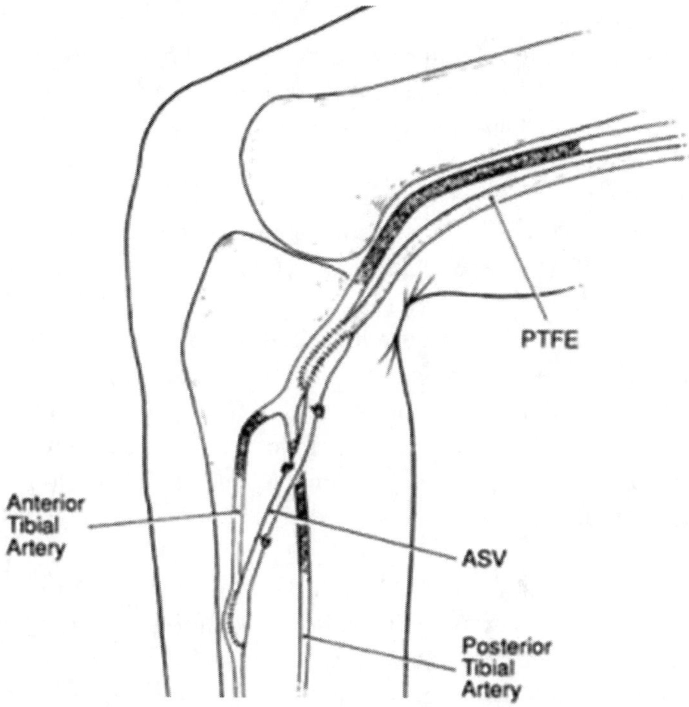

Figure 7.5 Diagram of composite jump bypass (source: Department of Vascular Surgery VUSCH).

Postoperatively, we monitor the blood supply to the limb, the skin's temperature and color, the pulse above the graft, and the movement and sensitivity of the acral parts. Postoperatively, we measure the ABI; if we suspect a bypass valve occlusion, we do not hesitate to perform a control angiography. After reconstruction due to severe ischemia, it is advisable to avoid compartment syndrome by administering mannitol; in case of progression, we choose fasciotomy. If trophic defects and gangrene are present, it is advisable not to intervene actively and wait for demarcation.

A good result is:

- if the anastomoses do not bleed
- if we palpate a pulsation under the distal anastomosis
- if pulsations are also present on the periphery of the lower limb.

In the ideal case, it is possible to perform intraoperative angiography (confirmation of the result of good bypass suturing) (Greenhalgh et al., 1994, Firt, 2006).

Pedal bypass

Pedal bypasses are arterial reconstructions that have a distal anastomosis located on the artery from the level of the ankles to the periphery of the leg (dorsalis pedis artery-DPA and its branches, distal part of the posterior tibial artery-PTA and its branches).

Veith (1986) first reported on patients who underwent limb salvage by suturing the bypass with a distal anastomosis sutured to the pedal artery. In Slovakia, the first more extensive set of these patients was published by Petrašovic et al. (1999).

These and crural bypasses are indicated only in patients with a compromised limb who have rest leg pain, trophic defects, or gangrene. However, not every defect is fully indicated for revascularization; minor defects (e.g., dry, apical) can heal over time with conservative treatment and regular bandages, even if it is a treatment of several months. Contraindications to pedal bypass are immobility of the patient, poor general condition, septic gangrene of the leg, and poor quoad vitam prognosis.

From the diagnostic and indication point of view, according to current knowledge, failure to visualize the pedal circulation is not considered a contraindication to surgery; it is enough if a Doppler signal is detected above the pedal artery. The definitive decision will be made only after the operational review. If DSA shows a collateral network without showing the main arteries, it can be assumed with a high probability that these are non-reconstructable conditions. On the contrary, if only a little of the contrast substance has leaked into the periphery, we can speak of underestimating the DSA finding. If a Doppler signal is present, operative revision is fully indicated.

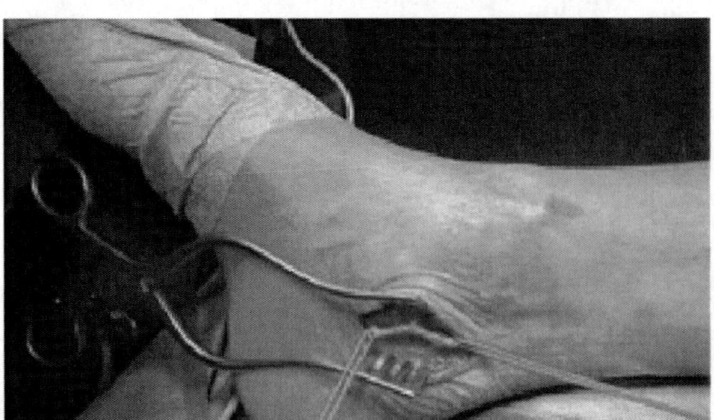

Figure 7.6 Posterior tibial artery before suturing the anastomosis (source: Department of Vascular Surgery VUSCH).

Operative procedure

We place the proximal anastomosis, most often on the popliteal artery, and if necessary, up to CFA using the sequential bypass. No statistically significant difference in patency and limb salvage has been demonstrated between femoropedal and popliteopedal bypasses, but shorter bypasses require fewer operative revisions for failed bypasses. The most common site of distal anastomosis is the dorsalis pedis artery, common plantar artery, or one of its branches, further lateral plantar artery (with a larger diameter but deeper placement), lateral tarsal artery, lateral anterior malleolar artery. There are no statistical differences in the long-term patency of bypasses on DPA or TPA and its branches. Artery diameters are often below 2 mm; Pomposelli indicates a pedal bypass for an artery with a diameter above 1 mm. We prepare gently, usually only the front wall of the artery; we use fine Fogarty catheters, microbulldogs, and intraluminal coronary shunts. Indicators of patency are sufficient return flow and minimal peripheral resistance during the instillation of heparin solution. Pedal artery endarterectomies are not recommended. We use monofilament fibers 6/0, 7/0, 8/0 to suture the anastomosis. The most suitable graft is the ipsilateral FSV or veins of the upper limb. Prosthetic materials have not proven themselves. A short bypass shortens the operating time; we run the tunnel subcutaneously along the medial surface of the foreleg. If acral amputations are necessary, we perform them in one stage. In the case of an extensive finding on the leg and a minimal outflow tract, a pedal bypass and a free muscle flap are possible; in contrast, the artery of the flap is sutured to the bypass and venous anastomosis to the posterior tibial vein, dorsalis pedis vein or GSV—the flap from the latissimus dorsi muscle, or rectus abdominis muscle.

The introduction of the pedal bypass methodology led to a decrease in primary (high) above-knee amputations from 41% to 5% and a decrease in all high amputations from 49% to 14%, long-term patency of 60-70% and 70-80% success in saving the limb, with a low postoperative mortality of around 2%.

Postoperative care - anticoagulation protocol

There are several algorithms for anticoagulant treatment in patients after bypass surgery.

In our workplace, the intravenous administration of 5000 IU of unfractionated heparin five minutes before clamping the artery has been proven effective. If necessary, we intravenously add 2,500-5,000 IU of heparin during the procedure. Postoperatively, in the ICU, we administer unfractionated heparin 4 x 5,000 IU s.c./24 hours and monitor the current state of hemocoagulation, possibly adjusting the dosage. If necessary, we use continuous heparinization at a dose of 30,000 IU/24 hours and monitor aPTT. Sometimes, we administer low molecular weight heparin (LMWH), which is also safe and effective. After discharge to outpatient care, the patient receives LMWH and is set on antiplatelet or anticoagulation therapy (optimally through the hematology clinic). Antiplatelet treatment reduces the incidence of graft occlusions by 1/3 (25% to 16%). Antithrombotic therapy reduces the risk of bypass occlusion by around 50% in 12 months. In high-risk patients, ticlopidine or clopidogrel 75 mg once daily is recommended. Clopidogrel is preferable to ticlopidine because of its side effects (leukopenia). Oral anticoagulants reduce the occurrence of ischemia but are associated with an increased risk of bleeding. The aspirin proves to be more beneficial for preventing occlusion of the bypass with a prosthesis, with a lower risk. Ariesen et al. (2005) derive antithrombotic therapy from the type of bypass: venous graft - oral anticoagulants, prosthetic graft - aspirin. Long-term LMWH therapy is not recommended, especially in patients with CLI, as it does not improve graft patency (Jivegard et al., 2005). Clagett et al. (2004) recommend a combination of aspirin and an anticoagulant at a high risk of bypass occlusion and possible limb loss.

Results of the operative solution

Graft patency and mortality

According to Firt, the immediate and long-term passability of the reconstruction is primarily determined by the quality of the bloodstream outlet. Proximal femoropopliteal bypass (FP bypass) for claudication with good outflow tract has an immediate patency rate of 96% or more; at five-year follow-up, patency remains in 80% of reconstructions. In patients in stages III. and IV. with a significantly affected outflow tract, the five-year patency is reduced to 55-65%.

Distal femoropopliteal bypasses have slightly worse results. Immediate passability is 90%, and five-year passability varies from 40-60%. The long-term results are worse in people with diabetes with rapid progression of atherosclerosis. In some patients, the defects healed, despite the later closure of the reconstruction. It is reported that the percentage of saved limbs is about 15% greater than the number of long-term patent bypasses.

Krajíček indicates the average patency of FP bypass during five years is 80% for venous bypass, 75% for bypass with prosthesis above the joint cleft, and 65% for bypass with prosthesis below the joint cleft. So, venous bypass above the cleft has about 1.7 times better patency than PTA. A study by Klinkert et al. (2004) demonstrated that the patency of FP bypasses sutured with vein graft is higher than bypasses constructed using expanded polytetrafluoroethylene (ePTFE). On the other hand, surgery is burdened with higher mortality and morbidity. We have to target the indication to a specific patient selectively. According to other large multicenter studies in patients with infrainguinal bypasses within one year, primary, primary-assisted, and secondary patency rates are 61%, 77%, and 80%, respectively.

Mortality of reconstructive procedures in the femoropopliteocrural area varies from 0-7.5%, with an average of 3.5%. Cardiopulmonary complications are the leading cause of death, as reconstructive surgeries are not age-limited.

Stenoses and graft occlusions

During the first year of follow-up, occlusion occurs in 10-20% of venous grafts, despite the autologous vein being most suitable for bypass in lower limb ischemia with a cumulative five-year patency of 60-70%. Long-term patency after revision (thrombectomy or thrombolysis) is 20-30%. Studies show that stenosed grafts have a three-fold higher risk of occlusion, and correcting stenosis is significant for long-term graft patency. Graft patency was evaluated in patients with CLI. During three years, 61 venous bypasses were sutured. There were seven deaths and six amputations during the monitored period. Overall one-year primary, primary-assisted, and secondary patency rates were 63%, 88%, and 88%, respectively. Cumulative annual limb salvage was 90%.

Other studies report annual cumulative primary, primary-assisted and secondary patency and limb salvage as follows: 67-68%, 74-77%, 84-100%, and 88-94%.

According to Berglund (2005), operative revisions were more frequent in venous graft patients than in ePTFE patients, and the outcomes of revised patients tended to get worse. However, it should be noted that the higher revision numbers in vein graft patients ultimately improved the overall success rate. Furthermore, they found that outcomes in patients with CLI treated with a graft (venous and ePTFE) over two years were similar and argued that ePTFE might be accepted in older patients with a shorter survival expectancy. In patients over 80 years of age, the survival results were better than expected, and the technical achievements were similar to the group with younger patients. The success rate was higher in patients with claudication than those with CLI.

Taylor et al. argue that the risk of occlusion during the second year of follow-up is low, and only one-year follow-up provides a benefit. Moody (1990) claims that a 6-month follow-up is sufficient because 94% of lesions manifest themselves during the first six postoperative months. Teo et al. (2001) point out that in their cohorts, 87% of stenoses or 88% of stenoses and occlusions were detected during the first year, as opposed to 65% or 67% seen during the first six months.

In 2006 Pereira et al. published a meta-analysis of 49 retrospective and 24 ongoing studies regarding FP bypasses. They evaluated proximal FP bypass (above the knee) with GSV or ePTFE and distal FP bypass (below the knee) sutured with GSV. It shows that the venous bypass above the knee has the highest primary patency, while the venous bypass sutured below the knee has the lowest within 27 months of suturing. The worst primary patency is with a bypass with a prosthesis sutured above the knee. Also, its secondary patency is the lowest (within 19 months), but the differences between individual bypasses are insignificant.

Complications of surgical treatment

They occur in 17-32%. They are characterized by the fact that they take place in the area of reconstructed arterial pathways. They have a local character and a dramatic course. The most significant risks are massive bleeding and closure of the reconstruction.

A common finding is swelling, which occurs on the 1st-3rd day after the operation. The cause may be an injury to the lymphatic system, deterioration of lymphatic drainage with impaired capillary permeability, or incipient venous thrombosis. Swelling subsides within 2-3 weeks.

Early postoperative complications

1, Bleeding – in 1-2% of cases. We monitor intraoperative and postoperative bleeding with a growing hematoma, bleeding from the wound, or increased output from Redon drains. We distinguish between local causes (from suture channels, the graft, the suture, and structures injured during dissection) and general causes (DIC, hyperfibrinolysis, consumption coagulopathy, and others). It is crucial to remove the detected malfunction. In case of greater perioperative bleeding, consumption of coagulation parameters and consumption bleeding may occur. No or minimal drainage from the drain may not yet rule out bleeding, as the drains may become occluded by coagulum or tissue detritus. We are guided by blood pressure, pulse, and blood count. More massive bleeding should be revised surgically, and the focus put mainly on the anastomoses area. Bleeding may also occur from interrupted retroperitoneal tissue or poorly ligated vessels.

2, Ischemia of the lower limbs: either from early reconstruction occlusion or distal embolization. Ischemia is manifested by pain, pallor, and coldness of the affected limb. Diagnostics consists of a clinical picture, USG, or CT examination.

Early occlusion is most often due to a technical error in the distal anastomosis area; it occurs in 1-2% of cases. The anastomosis may be narrowed, the intima may be dissected, the prosthesis may be bent or too long, or there may be poor drainage in the femoral area.

Distal embolization occurs if we do not remove the thrombus sufficiently from the prosthesis before its activation.

In surgical revision, we perform a thrombectomy and need to find out and solve the cause of the occlusion. A technical error in the distal anastomosis must be re-sutured; in case of poor drainage parameters, we add a femoropopliteal bypass to improve drainage.

3, Cardiac complications

They occur in 1-5% of cases, most often myocardial infarction, which is solved by PCI or CABG, rhythm disorders, hypertension, or heart failure. The complication is related to the extensive procedure's stress and the transfer of fluids in the postoperative period in connection with reperfusion.

4, Pulmonary complications

They occur in 7% of cases, the most common being postoperative bronchopneumonia. We treat it with intravenous antibiotics and expectorants.

5, Renal complications

Perioperative blood loss, reperfusion of the lower limbs, hypotension, and pre-existing renal insufficiency due to diabetes or vascular nephropathy play a role. They are manifested clinically by oliguria to anuria, requiring temporary dialysis. Acute renal failure after elective aortoiliac reconstructions occurs in 1-8% of cases.

Late postoperative complications

Reoperations for late complications are reported to be around 20%.

Occlusion of the reconstruction

It is the most common late complication; 15-30% of patients have an occlusion of the reconstruction within ten years. The most common cause is neointimal hyperplasia or progression of atherosclerosis (smokers) in the area of the anastomosis, but also pseudoaneurysms of the anastomosis, graft dilatation, and hypercoagulable state. Early occlusion occurs from the 3rd to the 30th postoperative day, typically based on incorrect indication or faulty surgical technique (graft breakage, improper placement, leaving adventitial strips, stretched graft, unsparing graft harvesting, and preservation technique, dissection of the distal intima, remaining thrombi, incorrect sutures, non-reversal position). Femoro-distal reconstructions, in which the quality of the outflow segment is not respected, should also be included here. The risk of these failures is the well-known fact that due to the immediate closure of the reconstruction, there is usually a significant worsening of the ischemia compared to the condition before the operation, which very often leads to the loss of the limb. This should be kept in mind when considering operations in the femoral-distal section without an explicit threat to the lower limb in functional IIa or IIb stages, according to Fontain. The prerequisite for the success of the reconstruction is the patency of at least one crural or pedal artery and the visualization of the pedal arch on angiography.

A significant technical predictor of early failure of primary patency is graft diameter < 3 mm; according to the study of Schantzer et al. (2007), primary patency was 85.7%, but for a vein larger than 3.5 mm, it was up to 93.2%. The primary patency of the composite vein was 84.1% compared with 92.2% for single-segment GSV. Suturing of longer grafts >60 cm had a primary patency rate of 53.7% compared to grafts <40 cm - 69.0%. Primary assisted and secondary patency was not affected by the length of the sutured graft. The treatment in case of graft closure is urgent surgical revision (thrombolysis or percutaneous interventional procedures are ineffective and contraindicated at this stage)!

Late occlusions appear after a period longer than two years, usually, a connection is found with the progression of the underlying obliterating disease.

According to the available literature, pseudoaneurysms in anastomoses occur in 1.7-23.8% of cases. Nowadays, the incidence is lower thanks to the improvement of surgical techniques and development in the field of sutures and prosthetic material. The most common localization is the femoral artery, and less often, the aorta, iliac arteries, and popliteal artery. Pseudoaneurysms arise as a result of insufficiency of the anastomosis suture. A pseudoaneurysm can lead to occlusion of the reconstruction, distal embolization, or bleeding. Diagnosis is by USG or CT AG. Treatment is surgical. The indication is a dimension above 2 cm or more than 50% of the graft. It is necessary to resect the pseudoaneurysm, replace it with a suitable interposit, and take the material for culture and sensitivity to rule out infection.

Infection is the most severe complication in vascular surgery. Local manifestations of infection of wounds and prostheses include common inflammatory manifestations (erythema, phlegmon, fluctuation, pain, fever, fistulation, purulent secretion, etc.) (Frankovičová et al., 1996). Staphylococcus epidermidis cause up to 50% of infectious complications. Infections have a subacute, chronic, and sometimes latent course. However, complications caused by staphylococcus aureus or gram-negative bacteria (E. coli, Pseudomonas, Proteus, Enterobacter, Bacteroides) are more acute, accompanied by destruction of tissues and vascular walls, and require urgent surgery. Infections located distally threaten the vitality of the limb. Centrally located aortic or iliac anastomosis infections represent a situation associated with a severe clinical condition and dramatic development requiring an urgent solution.

Risk factors for prosthesis infection include:

- repeated revisions
- presence of postoperative hematoma or seroma
- urgent aortobifemoral bypass

Even if the infection manifests itself after several years, it is assumed that the infection entered the wound during the operation; therefore, as a preventive measure, we prevent direct contact of the prosthesis with the skin already during the procedure (we cover the surgical field with foil), consistent hemostasis and drainage, avoiding concomitant procedures on the digestive tract. Clinically, the infection is manifested by bleeding, the occlusion of the reconstruction, and the rise of inflammatory markers in laboratory tests. From the imaging methods, CT, scintigraphy with labeled leukocytes, or PET CT can help; it will show the location of the infection. Surgically, the explantation of the entire prosthesis is fully indicated, with the subsequent restoration of blood flow to the limbs using an axillobifemoral bypass. Long-term treatment with

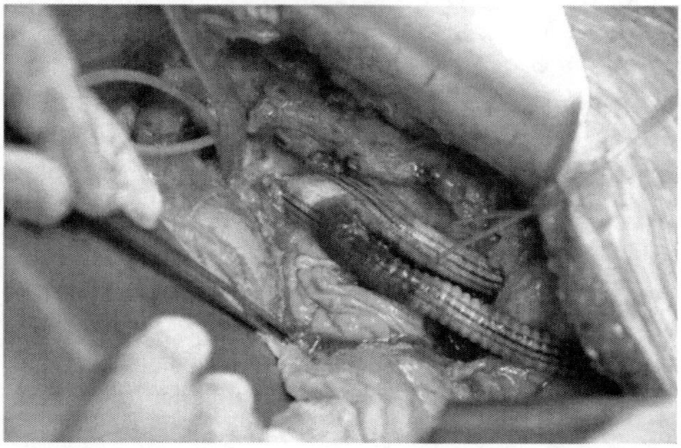

Figure 7.7 Graft infection in the groin (source: Department of Vascular Surgery VUSCH).

Table 7.2 Classification of prosthetic sepsis in vascular surgery according to Szilágyi and Samson (Štvrtinová et al., 2008)

grade I.: skin I. skin
grade II.: skin + subcutaneous tissue
II. skin + subcutaneous tissue
grade III.: vascular prosthesis
III. vascular prosthesis
IV. anastomosis + bleeding + septicemia

intravenous ATB is essential. Despite modern surgical procedures and intensive treatment, the mortality rate for prosthesis infection remains up to 50%.

References

ADAM, D.J. et al. Bypass versus angioplasty in severe ischemia of the leg (BASIL): a multicentre, randomized controlled trial. In Lancet, 2005, vol. 366, p. 1925–1934.

ALIMI, Y. S. et al. Efficacy of Viabahn in the treatment of severe superficial femoral artery lesions: which factors influence long-term patency? In Eur J Vasc Endovasc Surg, 2008, vol. 35, p. 346-352. 3. ALLIE, D. E. et al. 24-carat gold, 14-carat gold, or platinum standards in the treatment of critical limb ischemia: bypass surgery or endovascular intervention? In J Endovasc Ther, 2009, vol. 16, Suppl 1, p. I134-I146.

ALMAHAMEED, A. et al. Contemporary management of peripheral arterial disease: III. Endovascular and surgical management. In Cleveland Clinic Journal of Medicine, 2006, vol. 73 , Suppl., p. S45-S51.

AL-OMRAN, M. Use of interventional procedures for peripheral arterial occlusive disease in Ontario between 1991 and 1998: A population-based study. In Journal of Vascular Surgery, 2003, vol 38, p. 289-295.

Ariesen, M.J. et al.: On behalf of the Dutch Bypass Oral Anticoagulantsor Aspirin (BOA) Study Group. In Eur J Vasc Endovasc Surg, 2005, vol.30, p. 154-159.

ATAR, E. et al. Balloon angioplasty of popliteal and crural arteries in elderly with critical chronic limb ischemia. In Eur J Radiol, 2005, vol. 53, p. 287-92.

BALDWIN, Z. K. et al. Limb salvage after infrainguinal bypass graft failure. In J Vasc Surg, 2004, vol. 39, p. 951-957.

BECKER, H. et al. Management of Critical Limb Ischemia and Diabetic Foot. In Eur J Vasc Endovasc Surg, 2011,vol.42, no. 2, p. S4-S12.

Berglund, J. et al.: Long-term results ofabove knee femoro-popliteal bypass depend on indication for surgery and graft-material.In Eur J Vasc Endovasc Surg, 2005, vol. 29, p. 412-418.

CONRAD, M. F. et al. Intermediate results of percutaneous endovascular therapy of femoropopliteal occlusive disease: a contemporary series. In J Vasc Surg, 2006, vol. 44, p. 762–769.

CONTE, M. S. Results of PREVENT III: a multicenter, randomized trial of edifoligide for the prevention of vein graft failure in lower extremity bypass surgery. In J Vasc Surg, 2006, vol. 43, p. 742-751.

DIEHM, J. et al. Management of Critical Limb Ischaemia and Diabetic Foot. In Eur J Vasc Endovasc Surg, 2011, vol. 42, Suppl. 2, p. S34-S39.

DORMANDY, J. et al. Peripheral arterial occlusive disease: Clinical data for decision making. In Semin Vasc Surg, 1999, vol. 12, p. 93-162.

DORMANDY, J. A. et al. Management of peripheral disease (PAD). TASC Working Group, Transatlantic Inter-Society Consensus (TASC). In J Vasc Surg, 2000, vol. 31, p. S1-296.

FARRAJ, N. et al. One-year outcomes for recanalization of long superficial femoral artery chronic total occlusions with the Viabahn stent graft. In J Invasive Cardiol, 2009, vol. 21, p. 278-281.

FEINGLASS, J. et al. Postoperative and late survival outcomes after major amputation: findings from the Department of Veterans Affairs National Surgical Quality Improvement Program. In Surgery, 2001, vol. 130, p. 21-29.

FIRT, P. et al. Cévní chirurgie. In Karolinum, 2006.

FRANKOVIČOVÁ, M. et al.: Cievne komplikácie pri rekonštrukčnej chirurgii nohy, In Rozhledy v chirurgii, 1992, vol. 5, p. 251 – 253.

GREENBERG, D. et al. In-hospital costs of self-expanding nitinol stent implantation versus balloon angioplasty in the femoropopliteal artery (the VascuCoil Trial). In J Vasc Interv Radiol, 2004, vol. 15, p. 1065–1069.

GREENHALGH, R. M. et al. Vascular surgical techniques: An Atlas. In Saunders: London, 1994, p. 228-234.

HARTUNG, O. et al. Efficacy of Hemobahn in the treatment of superficial femoral artery lesions in patients with acute or critical ischemia: a comparative study with claudicants. In Eur J Vasc Endovasc Surg, 2005, vol. 3, p. 300-306.

HIRSCH, A. T. et al. ACC/AHA 2005 practice guidelines for the management of patients with the peripheral arterial disease (lower extremity, renal, mesenteric and abdominal aortic): a collaborative report from the American Association for Vascular Surgery/Society for Vascular Surgery, Society for Cardiovascular Angiography and Interventions, Society for Interventional Radiology, Society for Vascular Medicine and Biology, and the American College of Cardiology/ American Heart Association Task Force on Practice Guidelines

(Writing Committee to develop guidelines for the management of patients with peripheral arterial disease). In Circulation, 2005, vol. 113, no. 11, p. 463-654.

CHATURVEDI, S. The Seventh Report of the Joint National Committee in Prevention, Detection, Evaluation, and Treatment of High Blood Pressure (JNC 7): is it really practical? In Natl Med J India, 2004, vol. 17, no. 4, p. 227.

CHETTER, I. C. et al. Prospective analysis of quality of life in patients following infrainguinal reconstruction for chronic critical ischemia. In Br J Surg, 1998, vol. 85, p. 951-955.

Clagett, G.P. et al.: Antitrombotic therapy inperipheral arterial occlusive disease: The Seventh ACCP Conference onAntitrombotic and trombolytic Therapy. In Chest, 2004,vol.126, Suppl., p. 609S-626S.

Jivegard, L. et al.: Effects of Three monthsof Low Molecular Weight Heparin (dalteparin) Treatement After Bypass Surgeryfor Lower Limb Ischaemia-A Randomised Placebo-controlled Double BlindMulticentre Trial. In Eur J Vasc Endovasc Surg, 2005, vol.29, p. 190-198.

KAWAMURA, Y. et al. Nitinol stenting improves primary patency of the superficial femoral artery after percutaneous transluminal angioplasty in hemodialysis patients: a propensity-matched analysis. In J Vasc Surg, 2009, vol. 50, p. 1057-1062.

KEDORA, J. et al. Randomized comparison of percutaneous Viabahn stent grafts vs. prosthetic femoral-popliteal bypass in the treatment of superficial femoral arterial occlusive disease. In J Vasc Surg, 2007, vol. 45, p. 10-16.

KLINKERT, P. et al. Saphenous vein versus PTFE for above-knee femoropopliteal bypass. A review of the literature. In Eur J Vasc Endovasc Surg, 2004, vol. 27, p. 357–362.

KUDO, T. et al. Long-term outcomes and predictors of iliac angioplasty with selective stenting. In J Vasc Surg, 2005, vol. 42, p. 466–475.

KULLO, I. J. et al. Ethnic differences in peripheral arterial disease in the NHLBI Genetic Epidemiology Network of Arteriopathy (GENOA) study. In Vasc Med, 2003, vol. 8, no. 4, p. 237-242.

LAIRD, J. R. et al. Nitinol stent implantation versus balloon angioplasty for lesions in the superficial femoral artery and proximal popliteal artery: twelve-month results from the RESILIENT randomized trial. In Circ Cardiovasc Interv, 2010, vol. 3, p. 267-276.

LAMMER, J. Femoropopliteal artery obstruction: from the balloon to the graft. In Cardiovasc Intervent Radiol, 2001, vol. 24, p. 73-83

LEPÄNTALO, M. et al. Scandinavian Thrupass study Study Group. PTFE bypass or thru pass for superficial femoral artery occlusion? A randomized controlled trial. In Eur J Vasc Endovasc Surg, 2009, vol. 37, p. 578-584.

McQuade, K. et al. Randomized comparison of ePTFE/nitinol self-expanding stent graft vs. prosthetic femoral-popliteal bypass in the treatment of superficial femoral artery occlusive disease. In J Vasc Surg, 2009, vol. 49, p. 109-115, 116.

MEWISSEN, M. W. Self-expanding nitinol stents in the femoropopliteal segment: technique and mid-term results. In Tech Vasc Interv Radiol, 2004, vol. 7, p. 2-5.

Moody, P. et al.: Vein graft surveillanceimproves patency in femoropopliteal bypass. In Eur J VascSurg, 1990, vol.4, p.117-121.

NORGREN, L. et al. Inter-Society Consensus for the Management of Peripheral Arterial Disease (TASC II). In Eur J Vasc Endovasc Surg,2007, vol. 33, Suppl 1, p. S1-S75

PEREIRA, C. E. et al. Meta-analysis of femoropopliteal bypass grafts for lower extremity arterial insufficiency. In Journal of Vascular Surgery, 2006, vol. 44, no. 3, p. 510-517.

Petrasovic M, Belacek J, Holoman M. Pedálny bypass vliecbe uzáverovej choroby artérií dolných koncatín u diabetikov [Pedal bypassin the treatment of arterial occlusive disease of the lower extremities indiabetics]. Bratisl Lek Listy. 1999 Jun;100(6):312-6. Slovak. PMID: 10573646.

POBEHOVÁ, J. et al.: Porovnanie výsledkov chirurgickej a endovaskulárnej terapie u pacientov s periférnym artériovým ochorením dolných končatín vo femoropopliteálnej oblasti. In Rozhledy v chirurgii, 2014, vol. 93, no. 8, p. 416-423

48. RAJAGOPALAN, S. et al. Management of chronic critical limb ischemia. In Cardiol Clin, 2002, vol. 20, p. 535-545.

ROUX, A. et al. Early improvement in peripheral vascular tone following smoking cessation using nicotine replacement therapy: aortic wave reflection analysis. In Cardiology, 2010, vol. 117, no. 1, p. 37-43.

SABETI, S. et al. Primary patency of femoropopliteal arteries treated with nitinol versus stainless steel self-expanding stents: propensity score-adjusted analysis. In Radiology, 2004, vol. 232, p. 516-521.

SAXON, R. R. et al. Randomized, multicenter study comparing expanded PTFE-covered endoprosthesis placement with percutaneous transluminal angioplasty in the treatment of superficial femoral artery occlusive disease. In J Vasc Interv Radiol, 2008, vol. 19, p. 823-832.

SECOND EUROPEAN CONSENSUS DOCUMENT ON CHRONIC CRITICAL LEG ISCHEMIA. In Circulation, 1991, vol. 84, p. IV1-IV26.

SETACCI, C. Critical Limb Ischemia. New developments and perspectives. In Edizioni Minerva Medica, 2010

SHAMMAS, N. W. Epidemiology, classification, and modifiable risk factors of peripheral arterial disease. In Vasc Health Risk Manag, 2007, vol. 3, no. 2, p. 229-234.

Schantzer, A. et al.: Technical factorsaffecting autogenous vein graft failure: Observations from a largemulticenter trial. In Journal of Vascular Surgery, 2007, p. 1180-1190.

SCHRIJVER, A. M. et al. Hybrid procedures for peripheral obstructive disease. In J Cardiovasc Surg, 2010, vol. 51, p. 833-843.

SMEETS, L. et al. Outcome after occlusion of infrainguinal bypasses in the Dutch BOA study: comparison of amputation rate in venous and prosthetic grafts. In Eur J Vasc Endovasc Surg, 2005, vol. 30, p. 604-609.

ŠTVRTINOVÁ, V. et al. Choroby ciev. In Slovak Academic Press, 2008.

Teo, N.B. et al.: Effectiveness ofsurveillance of infrainguinal grafts. In Eur J Surg, 2001, vol.167, p. 605-609.

VEITH, F. J. et al. Six-year prospective multicenter randomized comparison of autologous saphenous vein and expanded polytetrafluoroethylene grafts in infrainguinal arterial reconstructions. In J Vasc Surg, 1986, vol. 3, p. 104-114.

Chapter 8

Extra-Anatomic Reconstructions

Jana Pobehová, MD*

Department of Vascular Surgery, East Slovak Institute of Cardiovascular Diseases, Košice, Slovakia

Abstract

Extra-anatomic reconstructions do not follow the anatomical pathways of the native artery. They were developed as a temporary solution to overcome emergencies for specific patients. The goal of treatment is to alleviate symptoms, reduce the risk of adverse cardiovascular events and preserve the function and vitality of the limbs. They include axillofemoral bypasses, iliofemoral bypasses, femorofemoral bypasses, and obturator bypasses. These reconstructions are effective in bypassing infected areas, avoiding infected areas, and in patients with a limited life expectancy.

Key Words: extraanatomical bypass, artery obliteration, infection, atherosclerosis

Arterial reconstructions cannot always be performed in such a way as to follow the anatomical course of the native artery. However, we always try to maintain sufficient inflow and outflow. It is not a conventional procedure, but often it is technically the last possible solution for obliterating artery disease. These reconstructions were developed as a "temporary" bridging of emergencies for specific patients.

The primary mechanism of peripheral artery disease (PAD) is atherosclerosis, in which plaque builds up inside the arterial wall. This clogs the vessel's lumen, causing a decrease in blood flow. This leads to a reduced supply of oxygen to the tissues. The vascular system's specific natural branching points and curvature

* Corresponding Author's Email: jana.pastvova@post.cz

In: Diabetic Foot
Editor: Martina Zavacká
ISBN: 979-8-89113-019-7

are more susceptible to atherosclerosis because of turbulent blood flow. Current understanding suggests that turbulent blood flow at very low tension compromises the integrity of the endothelium. Such hemodynamic changes seem to be associated with the development of focal atherosclerosis. Areas frequently affected include the aorta, coronary arteries, and carotids. Other causes of PAD include inflammatory vasculitis and non-inflammatory arteriopathies. The main risk factors for developing PAD are diabetes mellitus and smoking. The incidence of the disease increases with age; 20% of people over 60 have some degree of PAD.

PAD treatment aims to alleviate symptoms, reduce the risk of adverse cardiovascular events, and preserve limb function and vitality. Quitting smoking, modifying one's diet, and other healthy lifestyle changes significantly improve patient outcomes. The initial treatment approach is often balloon angioplasty with or without stenting to widen the arterial lumen and improve blood flow. Open surgical intervention is required to restore adequate blood flow to the lower extremities if endovascular access is impossible.

Before the development of extra-anatomic reconstructions, various arterial graft procedures were used to restore adequate blood flow around the area of obstruction. For example, in 1953, Freeman and Leeds published an article describing how the splenic artery was used to bypass the abdominal aorta. In 1960, cross-grafts between the common iliac arteries were described, and in 1961, bypasses from the thoracic aorta to the femoral artery were described. These procedures were successful in patients with unilateral occlusion but had limited use in patients at high surgical risk or with bilateral occlusion. In 1963, Blaisdell and Hall reported successfully performing the first axillofemoral bypass. In fact, they performed this procedure on three patients with high surgical risk and bilateral pelvic artery occlusive disease. In one of the patients, the reconstruction was performed using only local anesthesia, highlighting its utility in patients who could not tolerate general anesthesia. In addition, it provided a significant advantage over other procedures by avoiding an abdominal incision and aortic bifurcation.

In 1966, Sauvage and Wood modified the axillofemoral reconstruction procedure for bilateral pelvic artery occlusions and performed the first axillobifemoral bypass (AXbiFBG). In the original configuration of these grafts, the bifurcation was located at the level of the umbilicus. Flow rates differed in the ipsilateral and contralateral limbs, affecting the patency of these grafts. Subsequently, the configuration was changed so that the bifurcation occurred in the femoral region, and this configuration is still used today.

An indication for extra-anatomical reconstructions is, on the one hand, the general condition of the patient: patients with severe cardiac disease, severe lung disease, kidney failure, morbid obesity, malignant or systemic disease, with an expected patient survival of less than two years.

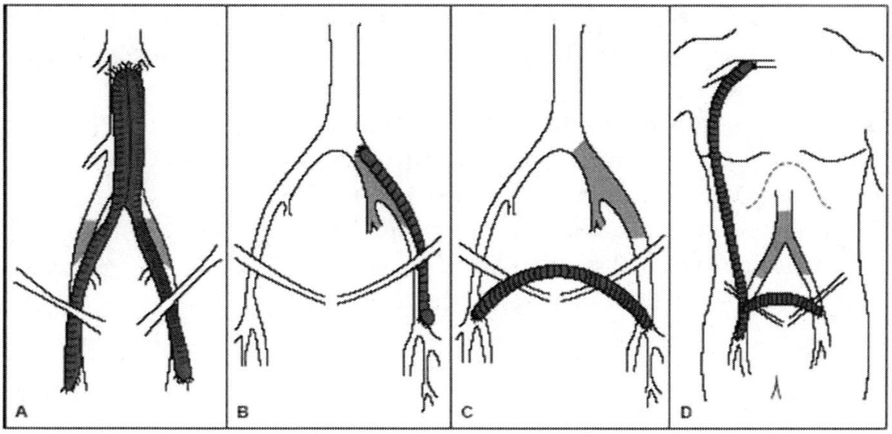

Figure 8.1 Types of extra-anatomic bypasses (source: Department of Vascular Surgery VUSCH).

Then, on the other hand, there are patients in whom it is necessary to bypass a particular anatomical area: scars, skin defects, colostomies, extensive abdominal hernias, conditions after local radiotherapy, or another group of patients with infections of vascular prostheses with a risk of bleeding, infected aneurysms, aortic dissections, or after nephrectomy.

One of the main complications of vascular surgery is prosthetic graft infection. The incidence of graft infection in the inguinal region varies between 1.3% and 6%. Postoperative amputation and mortality rates of 52% and 58% have been reported in association with surgical procedures for infections. Localized infection in the inguinal area can be treated with local methods, such as antibiotic therapy specific to culture and sensitivity from the surgical wound and inserting a new prosthesis with the removal of the infected part. Suppose bleeding or limb ischemia is present in association with graft thrombosis. In that case, the therapeutic protocol consists of systemic antibiotic therapy, removal of the infected graft, debridement of infected tissues, and reperfusion of the limbs. Extraanatomical revascularization is the most suitable surgical technique for overcoming limb ischemia in graft infection. After graft removal, either in situ implantation or extra-anatomic bypass methods must be performed. Graft removal and primary amputation are also permissible and can be life-saving in patients with severe bleeding, sepsis, or poor general condition. Axillofemoral bypass followed by immediate removal of the infected graft is indicated for aortic graft infections. The length of axillofemoral grafts also results in disadvantages such as susceptibility to thrombosis, proximity to the skin, and susceptibility to external pressure. On the contrary, the obturator bypass is considered an extra-anatomical bypass closest to the anatomical location, providing a permanent extra-anatomical reconstruction.

A separate group when extraanatomical reconstructions are indicated are hybrid procedures: implantation of stent grafts during EVAR/PEVAR, cervical debranching of supra-aortic branches, and cross-over bypass during a unilateral procedure at the iliac bloodstream.

It is essential to assess whether such a reconstruction will not cause a "steal phenomenon" - "stealing blood" from the original bloodstream to the detriment of the limb primarily supplied with it.

Iliofemoral and femorofemoral bypass

It is also known as a "cross-over" bypass; the first mention of its construction dates back to 1952 (Freeman and Leeds). The indication for suturing is typically one-sided occlusion of the pelvic bloodstream. Technically, the femoral arteries are secured infrainguinally, subcutaneously, or suprapubically (in Reitz's space). A bypass is performed in the shape of an inverted letter U or S.

We direct the recipient arteriotomy to the deep femoral artery, or we will add profundoplasty to it. Currently, a modified approach is widespread: the anastomosis in the tributary part is placed as proximal as possible to make the

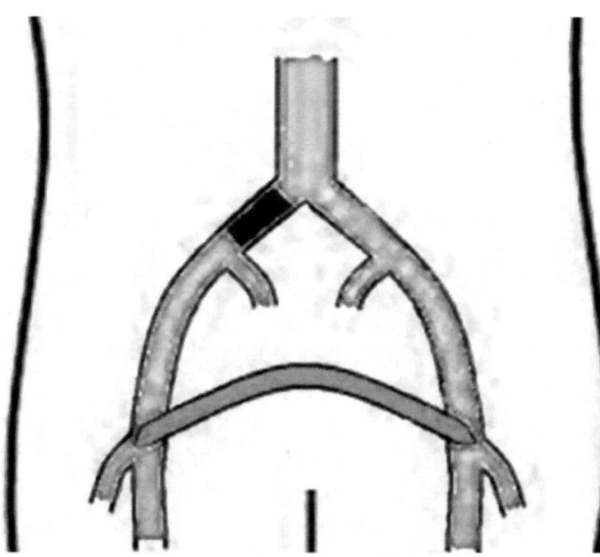

Figure 8.2 Femoro-femoral bypass "U shape" (source: Department of Vascular Surgery VUSCH).

blood flow more hemodynamically favorable. It is possible to suture up from the iliac artery to the retroperitoneum.

Obturator bypass

It was first constructed in 1962 by Shaw and Baue. Indications are infections, trophic changes, non-healing wounds in the groin, malignancy, tissue loss after radiation, and injuries. A prerequisite for successful reconstruction is the passability of the common and superficial femoral artery. The donor artery is usually the native artery in the pelvic area or an uninfected prosthesis segment. When conducting a bypass, we bypass the incriminated infrainguinal area through the obturator foramen. Subsequently, we construct a distal anastomosis in the unaffected place. It is necessary to avoid injury to the neurovascular bundle in the obturator foramen and to make a sufficiently spacious tunnel through the obturator fascia so that it does not mechanically close the reconstruction. Subsequently, it is necessary to solve the infectious process in the groin, explant the infected prosthesis, and remove necrotic masses.

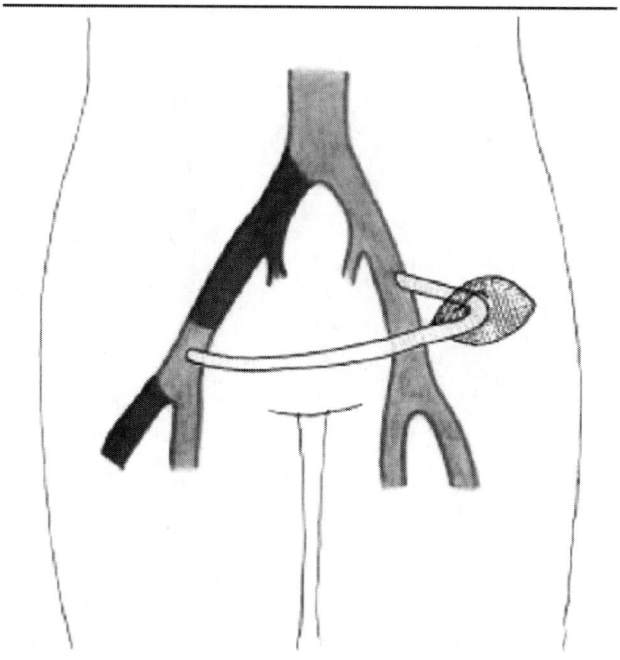

Figure 8.3 Ileo-femoral bypass (source: Department of Vascular Surgery VUSCH).

Obturator bypasses are often used in patients with infected pseudoaneurysms of femoral prostheses. Indications for its suturing include diffuse epidermoid carcinoma and radiation necrosis, secondary extensive soft tissue loss after trauma, and intense scar tissue presence. We sew the distal anastomosis to the femoral, popliteal, or profundal artery outside the infected area.

The primary purpose of the obturator bypass is to maintain the continuity of the new graft outside the infected area and to protect the graft from bacterial contamination. It is often necessary to use muscle flaps to preserve the graft's function and ensure effective wound healing. The angiosurgeon must be experienced and well-versed in the anatomical conditions in the given area. The most common complication is an obturator artery and nerve injury, passing through the obturator canal's lateral upper edge. Damage to the obturator nerve can lead to adduction and hip joint mobility limitation. Other complications include bladder rupture and pseudoaneurysm of the graft itself.

Literature reviews show that obturator bypass reconstructions are performed unilaterally. Cases of bilateral ones are rare.

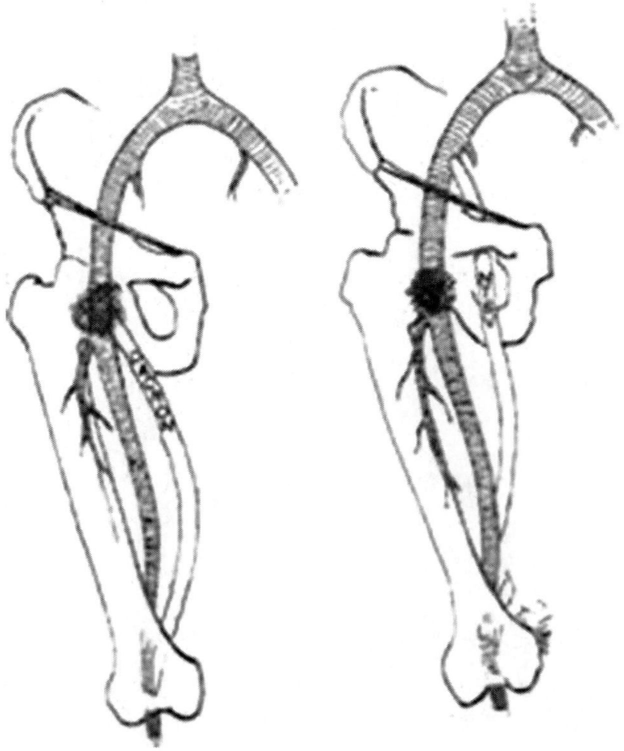

Figure 8.4 Obturator bypass (source: Department of Vascular Surgery VUSCH).

Axillofemoral bypass

This reconstruction was first carried out in 1963 by Blaisdell and Hally, USA. It is said to be the most common extraanatomical reconstruction. In 1966, Sauvage and Wood sutured an axillobifemoral bypass to both lower limbs. The most typical indication is infections in the aortoiliac region, with the impossibility of graft replacement. Technically, it is the suturing of the donor anastomosis to the axillary artery on the homolateral side, which is dissected in the sulcus deltoideopectoralis. For suturing, we pick the middle or medial third; we should avoid injury to the brachial plexus. The channel towards the limb is guided below the fascia or as a combination of sub and suprafascial space. However, they are more prone to repeated occlusions because they are extra-anatomical reconstructions.

The first axillofemoral bypass grafts were made of braided, unreinforced Dacron®, but there were problems with thrombosis due to graft compression during sleep. Kenney later demonstrated that using cast grafts with external reinforcement improved the four-year graft patency rate because they were practically incompressible. Burrell et al. (1982) compared the effectiveness of Dacron® versus polytetrafluoroethylene (PTFE) on graft patency and found no significant difference in patency rates. These conclusions were replicated and confirmed by Donaldson et al. in 1986.

Other attempts to prevent the formation of clots in the grafts involved various binding substances to the inner surface of the material (gelatin, collagen, and heparin). It is unclear whether these coated grafts affected the overall patency rate, as limited literature compares their performance.

For reconstruction today, we use a reinforced PTFE prosthesis of a suitable width, which protects the bypass from kinking. In the area near the infection, we choose an autologous vein graft or an allogeneic arterial graft.

Complications of extraanatomical reconstructions include:

- graft thrombosis
- graft infection
- seroma
- lesions of the brachial plexus
- steal syndrome

With advances in anesthesia and intensive care management, the postoperative mortality rate for aortobifemoral bypass is 3% to 5%, with an incidence of myocardial infarction of 2%. The long-term primary patency of aortobifemoral bypass is 80% to 92% after five years. 5-year primary patency rate for the axillofemoral bypass is 50% to 73%.

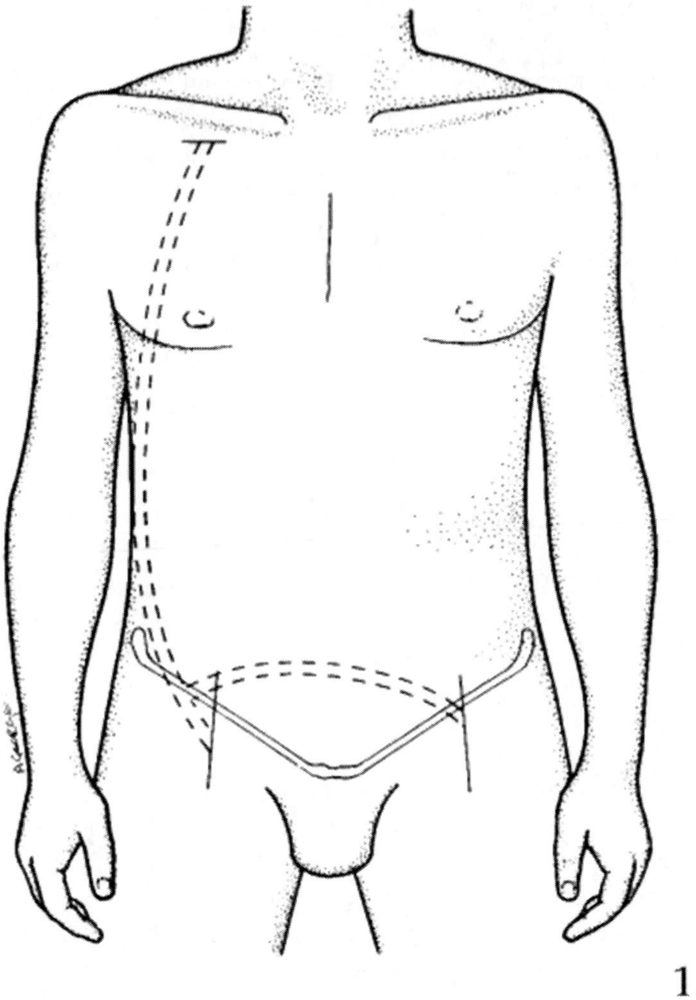

Figure 8.5 Axillobifemoral bypass (source: Department of Vascular Surgery VUSCH).

Complications are most likely to occur in the first 36 months after surgery, with an average of 21.5 months. Because of the potential for these serious complications, some have questioned the usefulness of these reconstructions. Despite the complication rate, the five-year rate of primary graft patency is reported to be between 54% and 80.4%. In patients who undergo thrombectomy, up to 97% can expect no further complications during the next five years.

Postoperative care of patients with extra-anatomic reconstruction includes using antithrombotic agents, especially in patients who require multiple reoperations to maintain graft patency. Evidence has shown that antiplatelet drugs such as aspirin may benefit patients with synthetic grafts. However, using warfarin was associated with an increased risk of bleeding. Patients should be routinely monitored for the recurrence of symptoms that indicate the development of thrombosis. Several available studies have shown no significant differences in primary patency in anticoagulation patients after extraanatomical bypass grafting versus no anticoagulation or anticoagulation with aspirin versus aspirin alone. Exploratory analyses identified an essential benefit of using anticoagulants in secondary patency for prosthetic bypasses, especially infrapopliteal ones.

In the 1990s, reports of improved results with sutured axillobifemoral bypass began to appear. Taylor et al. followed 184 patients who underwent axillounifemoral or axillobifemoral bypass using externally reinforced polytetrafluoroethylene (ePTFE) grafts with a diameter of 8 mm. The primary patency rate after five years was 71%.

Passman et al. retrospectively compared 108 patients who underwent axillofemoral bypass (AxFB) with 139 patients who underwent sutured

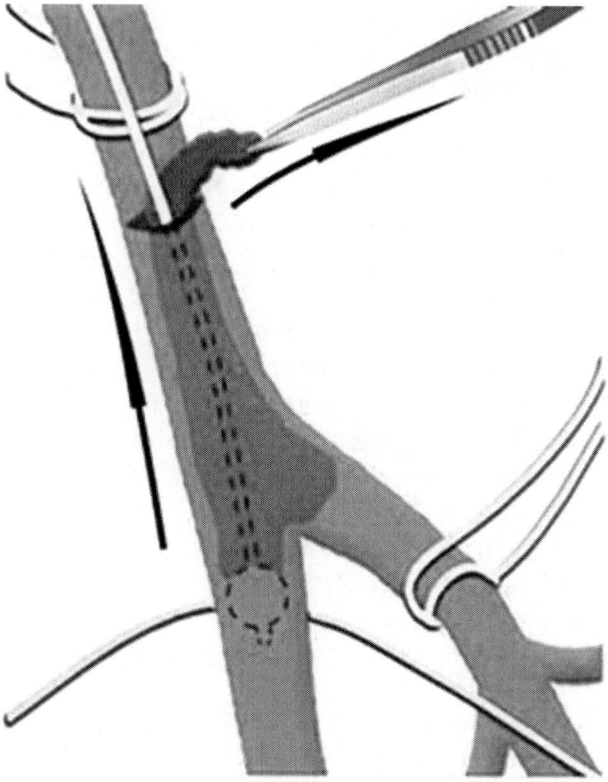

Figure 8.6 Scheme of bypass thrombectomy (source: Department of Vascular Surgery VUSCH).

aortobifemoral bypass (AoFB) and observed a 5-year primary patency rate of 74%. The difference between the AoFB and AxFB (80%) group was insignificant. Patient survival was lower in the AxFB group (45% versus 72%) primarily because it contained a more significant proportion of high-risk patients. However, the rate of major postoperative complications was significantly higher in the AoFB group (9.2% vs. 19.4%; $P < 0.05$).

Whether axillounifemoral (AxUFB) or axillobifemoral (AxBFB) bypass provides better patency has long been debated. Some early studies supported the idea that the AxBFB configuration would improve patency, possibly by increasing flow in the limb of the graft. More recent studies, however, have found no difference in patency between AxUFB and AxBFB. In addition, Martin and Katz observed that 60% of graft occlusions after AxFB occurs at the femorofemoral crossed limb. Therefore, AxBFB should be reserved for patients with bilateral disease.

In a study by Al Wahbi et al. published in September 2010, a total of 87 patients underwent extra-anatomic bypass (EABP), which included 28 (32%) femoral procedures and 59 (68%) axillary procedures. The median patient age at surgery was 67 years (range, 36–94 years), and gender distribution revealed a predominance of males (67%) over females (33%). Twenty-one patients (23%) underwent emergency surgery, and the remaining 66 (77%) were elective procedures. The indication for surgery was critical ischemia in 44 (51%) and severe claudication in 43 (49%). Patient comorbidities were found in similar frequencies in both groups. However, in patients with axillary surgery, there were significantly more patients with ASA > 3 (46 of 59 compared with 13 of 28; $P = 0.006$).

Postoperative complications included a total of 19 (21%) infections (17 axillary, 2 femoral), of which 12 (14%) were local skin infections (11 axillary, 1 femoral) and 7 (8%) graft infections (6 axillary, 1 femoral) . In six of them, the grafts had to be removed (5 axillary, 1 femoral). Early graft occlusion occurred in nine (10%) patients (7 axillary, 2 femoral). Thrombectomy was performed in all nine and was successful in four (3 axillary, 1 femoral). Revision surgery was performed in five (4 axillary, 1 femoral). Further surgery (excluding amputations) was performed in eight (7 axillary, 1 femoral). Eight (9%) patients died within 30 days of surgery (7 axillary, 1 femoral). Causes of death were cardiac ($n = 4$), septicemia ($n = 2$), and pneumonia ($n = 1$), and one cause was not recorded.

Primary patency rates for femoral versus axillary procedures at one month, 1, 3, and 5 years were 92% versus 93%, 69% versus 85%, 60% versus 72%, and 55% versus 67%, respectively. The survival rate was significantly lower in those who underwent axillary procedures ($P = 0.002$). Limb salvage rates for those who underwent femoral versus axillary procedures in this series were calculated as 100% versus 91%, 96% versus 84%, 96% versus 81%, and 92% versus 81% at one month, 1, 3, and 5 years, or there was no statistically significant difference in limb salvage rate for these two procedures (P = 0.124). A total of six patients required above-knee amputation, and five had a below-knee amputation, representing 12.6% of the 87 patients included in this study. Three of these 11 amputations (9 axillary, 2 femoral) followed the removal of the infected graft. Mortality in this subgroup of patients requiring amputation was 8%, 67%, 83%, and 83% at one month, 1, 3, and 5 years, respectively.

The authors emphasize that although there was a trend toward infection and early graft occlusion in patients undergoing axillary procedures, this was insignificant (P = 0.093). In addition, they found better primary patency outcomes but worse survival outcomes in patients with axillary procedures. In this series, the 5-year primary patency rates after femoral and axillary procedures were 55% and 65%, respectively. Older studies have shown comparable results after femoral procedures (52% to 83%) but worse long-term patency after axillary procedures (27% to 62%). They also found that five-year survival in this series was significantly higher after femoral procedures at 73% compared with 38% after axillary procedures. These data are favorable compared to other studies showing that 5-year survival is 42–80% for femoral procedures and 27–34% for axillary procedures. Worse survival after EABP is related to the adverse effects of advancing age, diabetes, hypertension, critical limb ischemia, and ischemic heart disease. The median age of all patients included in this series was greater than 65 years, and most patients had an ASA score of 3 or higher; therefore, the patients in this study were a high-risk population.

Regarding limb salvage rates, this series required major amputation in 11% of patients, consistent with previous studies reporting figures of 7.4–27%. Interestingly, further analysis of this subgroup revealed that 67% of patients who required amputation died within one year of their EABG.

Conclusion

Extra-anatomic bypass reconstructions have been shown to be effective in bypassing infected areas, avoiding infected areas, and in patients with limited life expectancy. An extraanatomical bypass can be used as a temporary reconstruction until the infected area has healed. With advances in anesthesia and critical care management, the postoperative mortality rate for aortobifemoral bypass surgery is 3% to 5%, with an incidence of myocardial infarction of 2%.

The long-term primary patency of aortofemoral bypass is 80% to 92% after five years. 5-year primary patency rate for the axillofemoral bypass is 50% to 73%. Several factors may have contributed to the improved outcomes with extra-anatomic bypass in our study and other recent series, including better anesthetic management, new antiplatelet and statin protocols, more specialized training and certification of vascular surgeons, and improvements in duplex ultrasound for graft monitoring. Nevertheless, extraanatomical bypasses have a fundamental role in managing selected patients.

References

Al-Wahbi A. Axillofemoral bypass with local anesthesia: a way forward to enable limb salvage in high-risk patients. Local Reg Anesth. 2010;3:129–132.

Burrell MJ, Wheeler JR, Gregory RT, Synder SO, Jr, Gayle RG, Mason MS. Axillofemoral bypass: a ten-year review. Ann Surg. 1982;195(6):796–799.

Donaldson MC, Louras JC, Bucknam CA. Axillofemoral bypass: a tool with a limited role. J Vasc Surg. 1986;3(5):757–763.

Dorffler-Melly J, Buller HR, Koopman MM, Prins MH. Antithrombotic agents for preventing thrombosis after infrainguinal arterial bypass surgery. Cochrane Database Syst Rev. 2003;(4): CD000536.

Freeman NE, Leeds FH. Resection of aneurysms of the abdominal aorta with anastomosis of the splenic to the left iliac artery. Surgery. 1953;34(6):1021–1031.

Geraghty AJ, Welch K. Antitrombotické činidlá na prevenciu trombózy po operácii infrainguinálneho arteriálneho bypassu. Databáza Cochrane Syst Rev. 2011;(6):CD000536.

Hardman RL, et al. Overview of classification systems in peripheral artery disease. Semin Intervent Radiol. 2014;31(4):378–388.

Jun Lee C, Lopez Rowe V. Axillofemoral Bypass. [Retrieved March 28, 2016];2015 Aug 13; from http://emedicine.medscape.com/article/1895225overview http://emedicine.medscape.com/article/1895225-overview.

Kempczinski R, Penn I. Upper extremity complications of axillofemoral grafts. Am J Surg. 1978;136(2):209–211.

Kenney DA, Sauvage LR, Wood SJ, Berger K, Davis CC, Smith JC, Rittenhouse EA, Hall DG, Mansfield PB. Comparison of noncrimped, externally supported (EXS) and crimped, nonsupported Dacron prostheses for axillofemoral and above-knee femoropopliteal bypass. Surgery. 1982;92(6):931–946.

Kullo IJ, Rooke TW. Clinical Practice. Peripheral Artery Disease. N Engl J Med. 2016;374(9):861–871.

Mannick JA, Nabseth DC. Axillofemoral bypass graft. A safe alternative to aortoiliac reconstruction. N Engl J Med. 1968;278(9):461–466.

Martin D, Katz SG. Axillofemoral bypass for aortoiliac occlusive disease. Am J Surg. 2000;180(2):100–103.

McCaughan JJ, Kahn SF. Cross-over Graft for Unilateral Occlusive Disease of the Ilio-Femoral Arteries. Ann Surg. 1960;151(1):26–28.

National Clinical Guideline Centre. London (UK): National Institute for Health and Clinical Excellence (NICE); 2012. Aug. Lower limb peripheral arterial disease: diagnosis and management; p. 12. (Clinical guideline; no. 147)

National Heart, Lung, and Blood Institute. [Retrieved March 27, 2016]; What is Peripheral Artery Disease? 2015 from https://www.nhlbi.nih.gov/health/health-topics/topics/pad#.

Passman MA, Taylor LM, Moneta GL, Edwards JM, Yeager RA, McConnell DB, Porter JM. Comparison of axillofemoral and aortofemoral bypass for aortoiliac occlusive disease. J Vasc Surg. 1996;23(2):263–269. Discussion 269–271.

Thompson JK, Strunk RS, Giglia JS. Bilateral obturator bypass for combined aortic and femorofemoral graft infection. J Vasc Surg. 2006;44:888–888.

Onoda M, Furutani A, Akiyama N, Morikage N, Yoshimura K, Hamano K. Infected aneurysms of bilateral deep femoral arteries due to Campylobacter fetus subspecies fetus. Ann Vasc Surg. 2008;22:476–480.

Shaw RS, Baue AE. Manažment sepsy komplikujúcej arteriálnu rekonštrukčnú chirurgiu. Chirurgia. 1963; 53 :75-86.

Skupina spoločnosti pre vaskulárnu chirurgiu dolných končatín na písanie pokynov. Conte MS, Pomposelli FB, Clair DG, Geraghty PJ, McKinsey JF a kol. Pokyny spoločnosti pre vaskulárnu chirurgiu pre aterosklerotickú okluzívnu chorobu dolných končatín: manažment asymptomatického ochorenia a klaudikácie. J Vasc Surg. 2015; 61 (3 dodatky):2S–41S.

Chapter 9

Limb Amputations

Peter Zavacký, MD*

Department of Surgery, Faculty of Medicine, Pavol Jozef Šafárik University in Košice and University Hospital, Košice, Slovakia

Abstract

We define amputation as removing a peripheral part of the body, including the softcover tissues, with disruption of the skeleton. Exarticulation removes the limbs at the level of the joints. Most frequently, amputations are performed for vascular causes, traumatic causes, the presence of osteosarcoma, and rarely in uncontrolled osteomyelitis or morphological defects. The leading cause of amputations is diabetic foot syndrome, which is also one of the most severe complications of diabetes.

Key Words: amputation, exarticulation, diabetic foot, infection

Amputation is defined as removing a peripheral body part, including the covering of soft tissues, with an interruption of the skeleton, which leads to a functional or cosmetic change with the possibility of further prosthetic treatment. In addition to it, we also know exarticulation. It differs from amputation in that the periphery is removed in the line of the joint. Exarticulations create residual limbs that are difficult to adapt to modern prostheses and often require soft tissue remodeling, myodesis, or myoplasty to sufficiently cover the bony prominences and thus ensure a comfortable fit of the prosthesis (Dungl, 2014).

The principles of amputations were established by the father of medicine, Hippocrates, 500 years BC:

---

* Corresponding Author's Email: peterzavacky963@gmail.com

In: Diabetic Foot
Editor: Martina Zavacká
ISBN: 979-8-89113-019-7

1. To remove diseased tissue
2. To reduce disability
3. To save a life

Modern flap amputations, including vascular ligation, using musculocutaneous flaps to create a soft cover, were first published by Lister and Brittain in 1837 (Dungl, 2014).

Most often, amputations are performed for vascular reasons, traumatic reasons, in the case of osteosarcoma, and rarely in the case of uncontrolled osteomyelitis, morphological defects, or a significant shortening of one of the limbs (Kolář et al. 2009). Nowadays, damage to the circulation in the lower limbs is a relatively serious issue, not only in the health sector but also in the social and economic sphere (Kolář et al. 2009). According to the WHO, the number of diabetes patients can be expected to increase to 300 million by 2025 (Kolář et al. 2009).

Approximately 40-60% of all lower limb amputations are performed in patients with diabetes. More than 85% of these amputations are caused by a foot ulcer that worsens to a deep infection or gangrene. The prevalence of diabetic foot ulcers is estimated at 3-8%. The complexity of these ulcers requires a multifactorial approach in which aggressive management of infection and ischemia is essential. For the same reason, a process-oriented approach is necessary for evaluating the prevention and management of diabetic foot. The healing rate of leg ulcers is unknown, except in specialized centers, where it ranges between 80-90%. The negative consequences of diabetic foot ulcers on quality of life include not only morbidity but also disability and premature mortality. The cost of ulcer healing is high and even higher for ulcers with amputation due to long-term hospitalization, rehabilitation, and the need for home care and social services for disabled patients. Therefore, one of the most important steps to reduce the cost of treating a diabetic foot is to avoid amputations. Recently, mortality after lower limb amputations has decreased to 5-10%. Generally, the higher the amputation, the higher the lethality, roughly 30% for above-the-knee amputations and 5% for below-the-knee amputations. Approximately 50% of deaths occur due to cardiovascular disease (Way et al. 1998).

The basic indications for amputations

1. Diseases of limb vessels

   Most often, these are amputations due to diabetic angiopathy, which leads to the development of diabetic gangrene associated with infection. Another common indication is acute or chronic arterial insufficiency. When preparing for amputation, multidisciplinary cooperation is necessary, where angiologists, angiosurgeons, and diabetologists work together to maintain the longest stump possible, thus ensuring the greatest possible mobility for the patient, who is often old and sick.

2. Trauma

   In the past, these amputations were relatively common, but nowadays, the only absolute indication is irreversible ischemia of traumatic or other etiology, thanks to the possibilities of microsurgery and vascular surgery.

3. Tumors

   Amputations are mainly performed for malignant tumors; they can also be used in rare cases for benign tumors in case of inappropriate localization or their size (jeopardizing the viability or function of the limb) or when there is a risk of their malignant transformation.

4. Infections

   These procedures are reserved for unmanageable acute sepsis caused by local infection or, on the contrary, for long-term infectious processes. For example, infection of the knee joint replacement can also be a borderline case. With these causes, the patient's life is at risk, so these amputations are performed to save a life.

5. Congenital anomalies

   Amputations only occur if the malformation of the limb is to such an extent that it is impossible to equip it with orthotics or prosthetics.

6. Necrosis

   It also includes necrosis due to physical effects such as burns, electric shocks, frostbite, etc., when it is possible to decide on the level of amputation only after the necrotic focus has been defined.

7. Skin condition or soft tissue defect

   Considering the possibilities of microsurgery and vascular surgery, this indication is relative.

8. Nervous diseases and injuries

   Amputations due to neuropathies occur when trophic ulcers appear, which lead to secondary infection, which can lead to a threat to the limb or a danger to the patient's life. Exceptionally, amputations are indicated for people with paraplegia because they help maintain the patient's balance in a wheelchair and, at the same time, act as a preventive measure against pressure ulcers due to the distribution of momentum (Sosna et al. 2001, Kubeš 2005, Brozmanová et al. 1990).

The leading cause of amputations is diabetic foot syndrome, which is also one of the most severe complications of diabetes. According to WHO, diabetic foot syndrome is defined as ulceration and the destruction of foot tissues associated with neuropathy, angiopathy, and infection. Due to its frequent recurrences, this diagnosis is considered lifelong (Rybka 2007).

Risk factors for ulceration are previous ulcerations or amputations, sensorimotor neuropathy, injuries (due to falls, walking barefoot, inappropriate footwear), biomechanical factors (reduced joint mobility, leg deformities, hyperkeratosis), ischemic disease of lower limbs, social and economic factors (low social level, insufficient health care) (Jirkovská 2006).

40-70% of all lower limb amputations are performed on people with diabetes (Rybka 2007). Almost half of those with diabetes are hospitalized because of diabetic foot syndrome. Although gangrene and lower limb defects precede amputations, these patients' hospitalization is relatively long, not to mention the significant financial costs incurred for their treatment (Rybka 2007).

Amputation is performed using an open or closed technique. With the open technique, the amputation wound is not primarily closed; one more operation is needed to create a stump. By amputation, we can relieve pain and change the patient's health.

Types of amputations by cause

1. primary – a condition when the amputation was caused by trauma; replantation is possible if the amputated part is available or the amputation stump is treated.
2. secondary – a condition when a life-threatening condition occurs, caused by necrosis, purulent processes with overall intoxication of the organism. Since conservative treatment procedures have failed, it is necessary to proceed with amputation.
3. tertiary (postponed) – in case of polytrauma, when it is necessary to ensure essential vital functions, amputation is possible only after the condition has stabilized.

   An amputation requires an individual approach, evaluation of the patient's overall condition and limb, the height of amputation, the patient's occupational classification, and consultation with a prosthetics technician.

Types of amputations (according to the used method)

1. guillotine (circular, open)

   First, the skin is cut in a circular motion and allowed to retract. Where the retraction ends, the muscles are cut and retracted again. At the end of the retraction, the bone is cut. Before closure, the stump must be adjusted for the prosthesis.

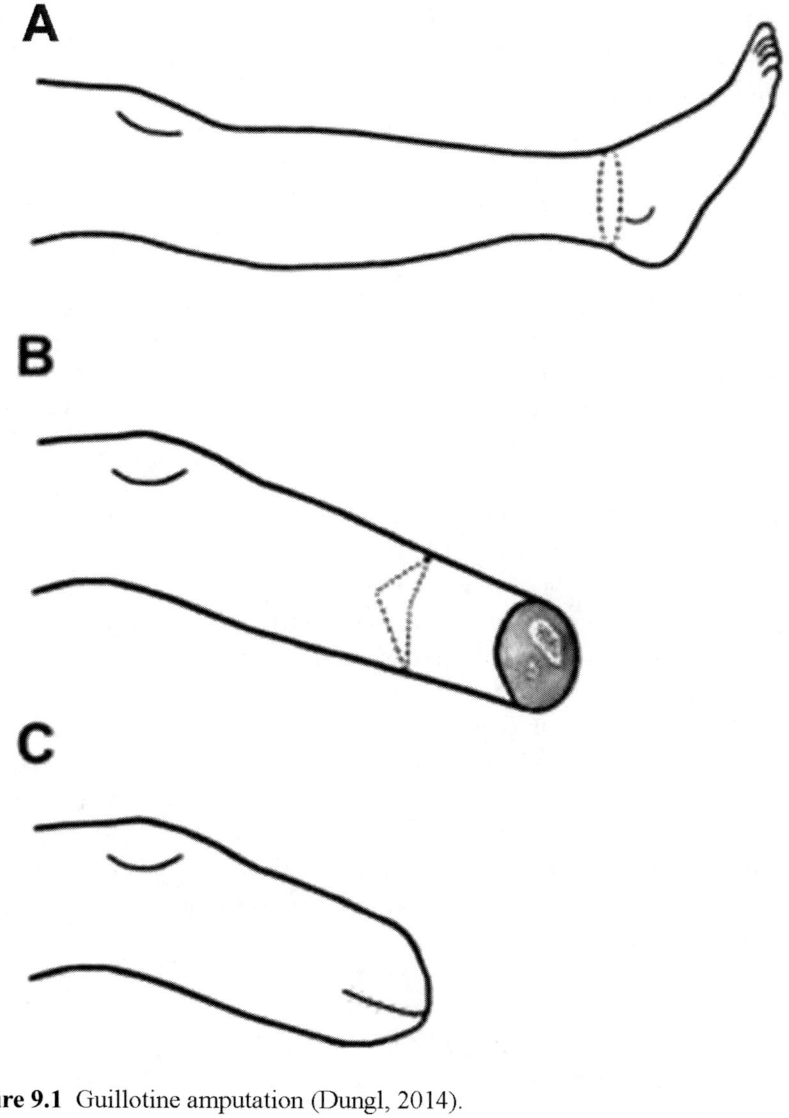

Figure 9.1 Guillotine amputation (Dungl, 2014).

2. flap amputation (open and closed technique)

   This is a standard procedure when we create skin flaps, invert them, and sew them together. We must plan the placement of the flaps so that all pathological tissue is removed and the skeleton is interrupted at the planned height. We only interrupt it at the end, after the skin and muscle flaps have been created. We strive to preserve the motility of the stump by myoplasty (we connect the muscles of a particular group with their antagonists - most often flexors and extensors, except the fingers!), or myodesis (reinsertion - we create a new muscle insertion, e.g., adductors of the thigh).

We place the amputation scar outside the footing surface of the stump. We pay special attention to the treatment of nerves; it prevents amputation neuroma. The most ideal seems to be withdrawal and sharp interruption with gradual retraction.

Types of upper extremity amputations (according to location):

1. finger amputations (replaced cosmetically)
2. amputations in the middle of the metacarpal bones (replaced cosmetically)
3. exarticulation in the wrist (performed rarely due to the complicated creation of the prosthesis)
4. amputation of the forearm (assessed according to the level of the disability)
5. amputation of the forearm stump, according to Krukenberg (the muscles between the two bones in the forearm, the radius, and the ulna, are cut, thus creating a "clap" that performs a shearing movement)
6. exarticulation in the elbow (it has good conditions for the creation of a prosthetic replacement)
7. amputation in the arm (assessed according to the level of disability)
8. exarticulation in the shoulder joint (the prosthesis is more of a cosmetic issue)
9. amputation of part of the scapula and clavicle
10. amputation of the entire shoulder girdle (the whole scapula, clavicle, and scapular muscle are removed, and only the trunk remains, the prosthesis is a cosmetic matter).

Lower limb amputations:
Hemicorporectomy – removal of the entire pelvic girdle. In this type of amputation, part or all of the pelvic girdle is removed along with the sacrum. Providing a stoma solution for the GIT and excretory tract is necessary. Prosthetic treatment is complicated but essential to ensure the mechanical protection of the organs in the abdominal cavity (Kubeš 2005, Brozmanová et al. 1990).

Hemipelvectomy – removal of a lower limb with half of the pelvis. Indications are mainly malignant tumors of the lower limb or pelvis and cases where the patient's life is at risk (Way et al. 1998, Křivánek, Eis 1972). During a hemipelvectomy, the entire lower limb with the adjacent part of the pelvic bone is removed. If the entire pelvic bone is removed, it is a radical hemipelvectomy. In a conservative type of operation, the part of the pelvic bone that adjoins the sacrum is preserved. Internal hemipelvectomy is a procedure

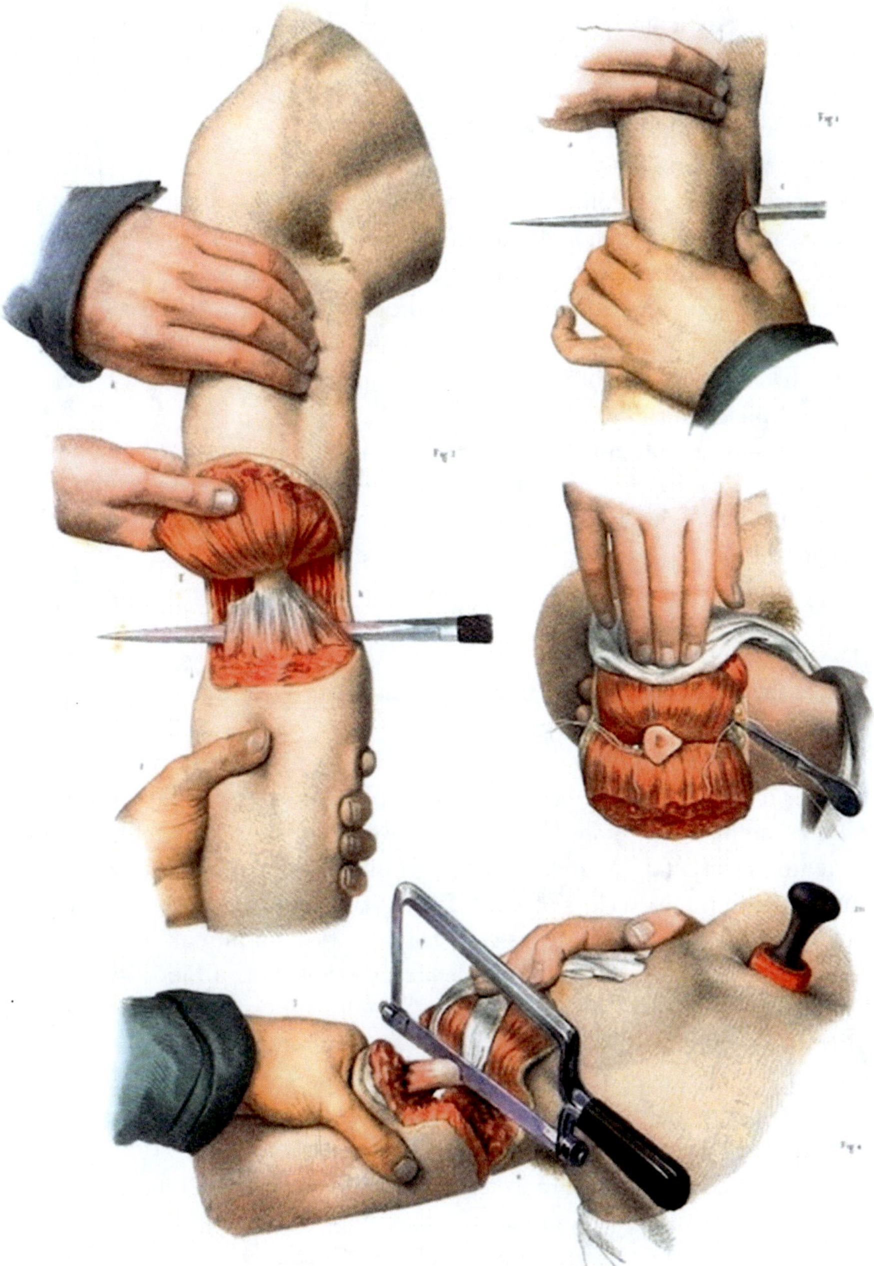

Figure 9.2 Amputation of the upper limb (source: www.etsy.com).

in which a particular part of the pelvic bone and the associated muscles are removed, but the lower limb is preserved (Kubeš 2005, Way et al. 1998). With this amputation, no weight-bearing stump is formed; therefore, prosthetic treatment is complicated (Křivánek, Eis 1972, Brozmanová et al. 1990).

Exarticulation of the hip joint - with removing the acetabular cartilage for sequestration. Indications for this type of amputation are high-reaching gangrene, severe infections, and tumors of the thigh or lower femur (Zeman et al. 2004, Way et al. 1998). In the case of exarticulation in the hip joint, a weight-bearing stump is formed in the area of the ischial tuberosity. Prosthetics using a pelvis is possible, and the entire lower limb is cosmetically replaced. Most patients cannot be rehabilitated, and walking is problematic (Way et al. 1998, Brozmanová et al. 1990, Křivánek, Eis 1972).

Femoral amputation – is the most common. This type of amputation is indicated in the case of necrosis in the area of the foreleg, in severe infections, and in patients who are not likely to walk in the future (Zeman et al. 2004). Amputation is most often performed at three levels:

1. above the condyles
2. at the border of the middle and distal third
3. at the border of the proximal and middle third (Zeman et al. 2004)

The main advantage of femoral amputation is the high probability of healing, but the disadvantage is the low number of walking patients - roughly only 40% of amputees (Zeman et al. 2004). Adductor myodesis is used laterally in femoral amputations through the top of the bony stump. The flexors are sutured with the extensors through the top of the stump using the myoplastic method. However, myoplasty is a contraindication for amputations performed for vascular reasons due to the possible deterioration of blood supply to the thigh muscles (Kubeš 2005). .In general, the longer the stump, the more powerful it can be. However, if the stumps are too long, it can complicate prosthesis manufacturing and thus decrease their performance. On the contrary, a short amputation stump has almost no functional value because it is impossible to carry out movement in the hip joint. In addition, the stump takes on a flexion and abduction contracture, and prosthetics are also more demanding (Křivánek, Eis 1972, Brozmanová et al. 1990). In the lower amputations, we include Gritti and Callender amputations. In Callender amputation, the surgical procedure is performed just above the condyles of the femoral bone, and the antagonists of the femoral muscles are sutured together. In Gritti amputations, we distinguish two types, short and long Gritti, depending on the height of the resection of the femur. In short Gritti, the femur is usually cut above the condyles, and the rest of the kneecap is folded over the stump after removing the cartilage. Today, however, the long Gritti is used more often when the femur is cut at the epiphysis and diaphysis junctions. The operative procedure is the same for both; it is essentially an osteoplastic method (Křivánek, Eis 1972, Brozmanová et al.

Exarticulation in the knee joint - a high-quality stump remains for good prosthesis retention. This type of amputation is mainly indicated for young men and brings several advantages:

1. provides a high-quality weight-bearing stump
2. the swing phase of walking is preserved due to the preservation of the long lever of the thigh muscles
3. the stump provides a firm and good hold of the femoral socket of the prosthesis
4. such a sufficiently long stump facilitates sitting and standing up and helps maintain balance (Zeman et al. 2004, Kubeš 2005). The most common method for exarticulation is the resection of the condyles in the transverse plane and firm fixation of the patella to the resected line. Submerged tension screws or Zahradníček's nails are then used for fixation. In this way, the patella with the skin cover becomes a footing surface, and the function of the thigh muscles is preserved (Kubeš 2005).

   Foreleg amputation - it is the second most frequently performed type of amputation. Primary healing can be expected in almost 80-100% (Kubeš 2005). In case of amputation in the area of the foreleg, it is essential that the resection of the fibula is always more proximal than the resection of the tibia and that the anterior edge of the tibia is abraded at the resection site. This will ensure the correct formation of the stump and, at the same time, prevent skin bruises in place of these prominences (Kubeš 2005, Way et al. 1998). A short, medium, or long fore-knee stump can be preserved in case of fore-knee amputation. However, if the knee stump is too short, it creates a short lever, which is not very suitable for controlling the prosthesis, and in addition, it has a great tendency to develop a flexion contracture (Brozmanová et al. 1990). Rehabilitation tends to be relatively successful. Roughly 90% of patients learn to walk with a prosthesis. However, rehabilitation success depends on the overall mobility of the patient before surgery and the quality of preoperative rehabilitation. Less than 15% of patients who were immobile before amputation are successfully rehabilitated (Zeman et al. 2004, Way et al. 1998).

Syme, Chopart, Lisfrank, Boyd, and other leg amputations

Amputations in this part of the leg must create a stump (suitable for stepping on) and leave room for the leg prosthesis joint. Syme, Pirogov, and Boyd

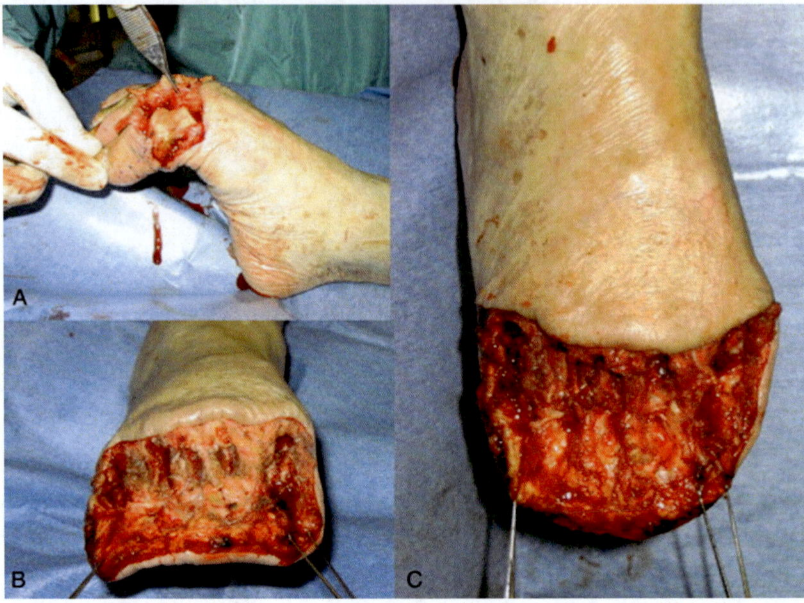

Figure 9.3 Open flap amputation (source: Department of Vascular Surgery VUSCH).

amputations are performed (Kubeš 2005). Syme amputation is essentially a disarticulation in the ankle joint. The tibia and fibula must be resected perpendicular to the stepping plane, just above the tibial cartilage. In addition, a subperiosteal resection of the calcaneal flap is also necessary, which must be firmly fixed until healing is completed. Indications are usually tarsal injuries with good blood supply to the heel and ankle (Kubeš 2005, Way et al. 1998). Pirogov and Boyd's amputations are quite complicated and, therefore, not recommended nowadays. In Pirogov amputation, all the leg bones are removed except for 3/4 of the heel bone, which, together with the Achilles tendon, is attached to the distal part of the tibia and thus creates a stump (Kubeš 2005, Sosna et al. 2001). With amputation in this area, the limb is shortened by only a few centimeters. A prosthesis is unnecessary and only a cosmetic replacement (Way et al. 1998).

Chopart and Lisfranc amputation

In Chopart amputation, the bones in the talonavicular and calcaneocuboid joints are separated during the procedure. It is essentially an exarticulation (Kubeš 2005, Sosna et al. 2001). In Lisfranc amputation, tarsometatarsal exarticulation occurs (Kubeš 2005). Both types of amputations are not very popular due to the possibility of an equinox leg deformity with insufficient weight bearing and a problematic scar (Kubeš 2005, Way et al. 1998).

Transmetatarsal amputation

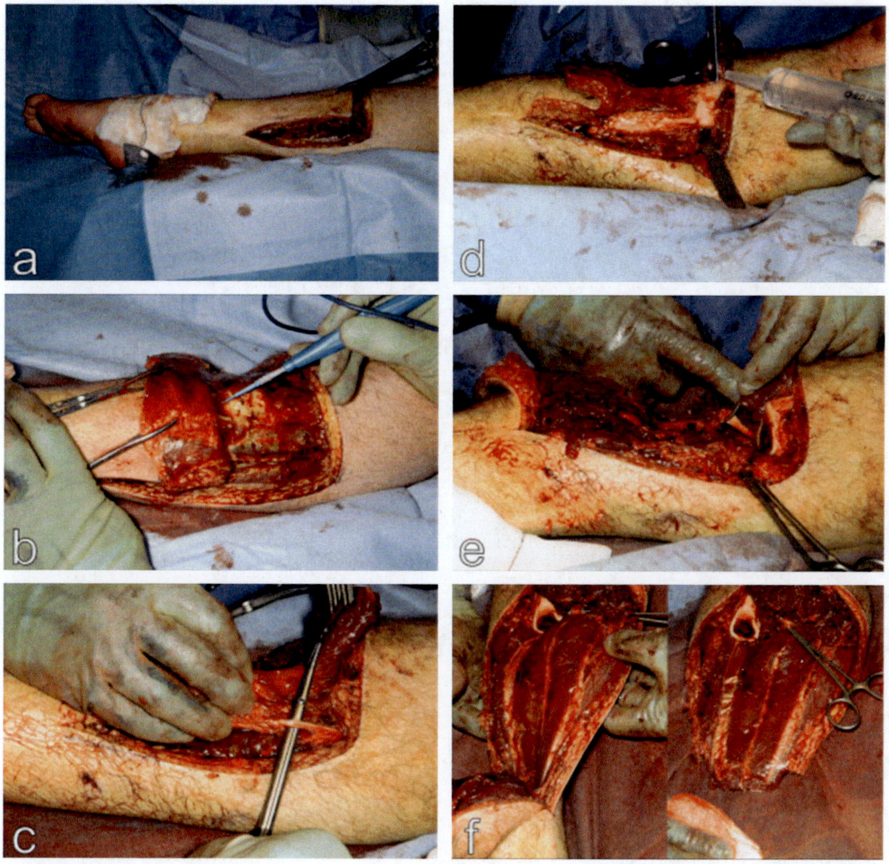

Figure 9.4 Foreleg amputation (source: Department of Vascular Surgery VUSCH).

Indications for amputation are gangrene of several fingers with or without soft tissue infection or osteomyelitis. The plantar skin must be healthy, and there must be no signs of spread of infection to the foot (Way et al. 1998). In transmetatarsal amputation, it is necessary to carry out the resection just above the metatarsal heads. This type of amputation allows for maintaining normal weight distribution. Walking and movement are usually smooth without increased energy demand. A special prosthesis is unnecessary, but the footwear must be specially modified, using sheep's wool or specially shaped foam (Way et al. 1998, Kubeš 2005).

Toe amputation and toe amputation with a partial metatarsal amputation

Indications for amputation are gangrene, infection, neuropathic ulceration, and osteomyelitis affecting the middle and distal phalanx. Overall, it can be said that more than 2/3 of the toe and metatarsal amputations are indicated

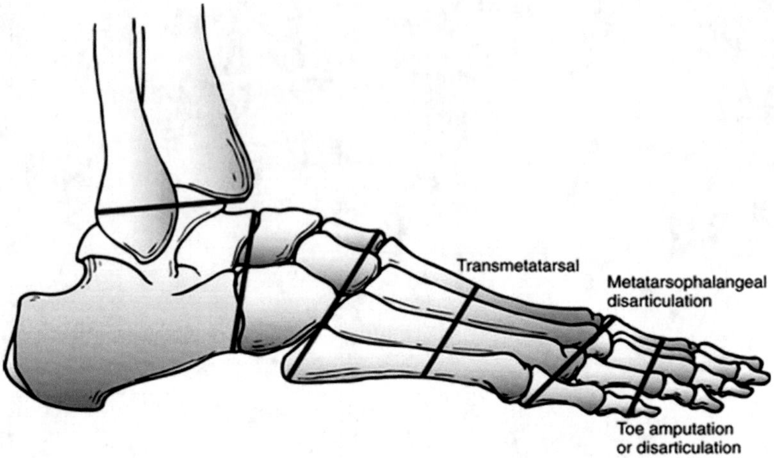

Figure 9.5 Foot amputations (source: www.musculosceletalkey.com).

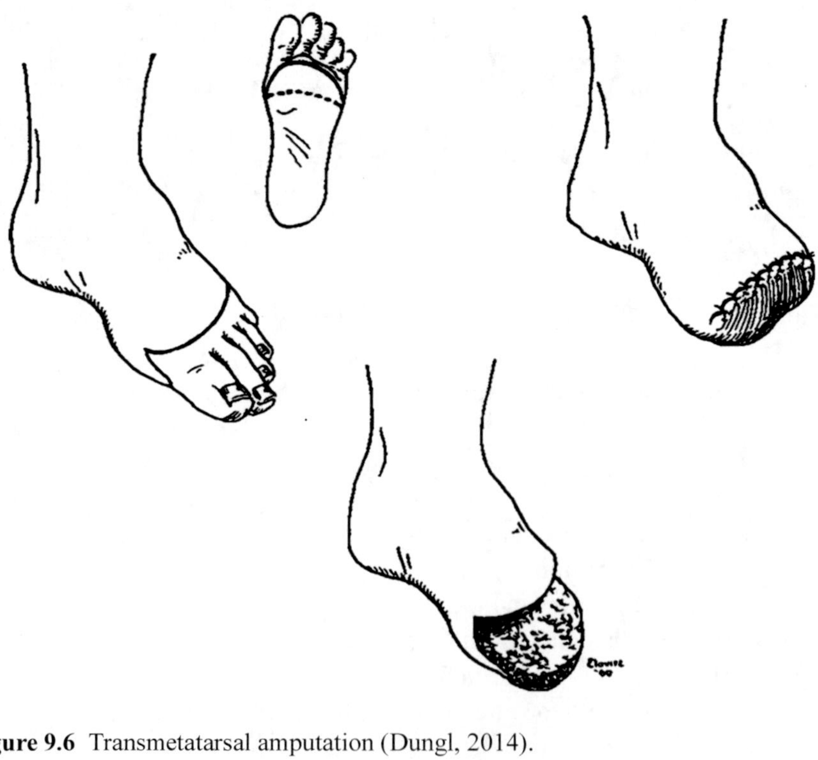

Figure 9.6 Transmetatarsal amputation (Dungl, 2014).

for diabetes mellitus (Way et al. 1998). In toe amputation with partial metatarsal amputation, the toe and metatarsal head, or two adjacent toes, are removed. During amputation, the vascular supply of the area must be in good condition (Way et al. 1998). In dry and non-infected gangrene, it is possible to carry out auto-amputation. In this method, epithelization and subsequent spontaneous detachment of the finger occurs. This way, a clean stump is created, localized in the most distal place. The only disadvantage of this process is that it can take up to several months (Way et al. 1998).

Amputation of the big toe and part of the involved metatarsal causes walking and running problems due to weight-bearing instability and lack of support in the rebound phase. For this reason, it is advisable to secure the position of the sesamoid bones by preserving even a tiny part of the phalanx base. Suturing of extensors and flexors is also suitable (Way et al. 1998, Kubeš 2005).

A valgus thumb can occur when the second toe is amputated (Kubeš 2005). With these amputations, there is no cosmetic deformation. Therefore a special prosthesis is unnecessary; it is enough to use only a prosthetic filling for shoes (Way et al. 1998, Kubeš 2005). Contraindications to toe amputation include unclear demarcation of the area, infection at the level of the metatarsals, and ischemia in the metatarsal (Way et al. 1998).

During amputations, we proceed as follows:

1. Bleeding protection: if possible, a tourniquet is usually used to clarify the operative field better. It is not used for vascular indications.
2. Cut through the skin: it is interrupted as distally as possible, as it tends to retract by about a third. In addition, it is necessary to pay attention to the shape and location of the scar, which essentially depends on the level and type of amputation.
3. Cutting of soft parts (muscles) and periosteum: during amputation, it is crucial to leave as much of the most efficient muscle as possible because it is necessary to consider that the muscle will retract and atrophy. Based on the skin and muscle flaps, amputations can be single-flap or double-flap. If it is possible to cover the bone stump with muscle attachments, it is called tendoplastic amputation (myodesis). With this type of amputation, a new muscle attachment is created, which allows the preservation of the original function and, at the same time, prevents contractures. Suppose the bone stump is covered by muscle tissue; then the opposite muscle groups (most often flexors and extensors) are stitched together under slight tension. In that case, we speak of a myoplastic amputation.
4. Sawing the bone: an oscillating saw is used for the osteotomy. After the bone is cut, the bone stump is covered with periosteum with bone lamellae or a part of the bone that comes from the removed peripheral stump

can be attached to the cut surface of the bone. Bony protuberances should be beveled.

5. Treatment of vessels and nerves: the vessels are cut in isolation and treated by ligation. Even before the wound is closed, the tourniquet is released, and the bleeding is stopped. Thorough hemostasis is a prerequisite for good healing of the amputated leg. As for the nerves, a technique is used in which the nerves are gently pulled out of the operative field and sharply cut.
6. Closure of the surgical wound using drainage: Redon drainage is inserted into the wound for 48-72 hours. Preventing the formation of a hematoma is very important because, in the event of its formation, the tissues are exposed to tension, and this is both the cause of pain and, on the other hand, it prevents healing with the potential risk of infection (Sosna et al. 2001, Kubeš 2005, Brozmanová et al. 1990).

Edema prevention by elevating the operated limb using an adjustable bed is very important. We must avoid flexion that would lead to flexion contractures. Sutures are removed between the 10th and 14th day, assuming trouble-free healing. The stump is gradually bandaged from its apex in the proximal direction using an elastic bandage to shape it properly (Sosna et al. 2001).

Amputation with creating a high-quality stump is sometimes the only possible solution in treating severely dilacerated limbs and their parts, without prospects for restoring circulation and function. A fundamental requirement is the creation of a painless stump and preserving joint mobility with sufficient soft tissue coverage. Scars must not interfere with the function of the prosthesis. Peripheral nerves must be treated so that the amputation neurons are not irritated by the touch or pressure of the prosthesis (Maňák, 2005). The stump of the humerus should be at least 12 cm long, and the stump of the forearm at least 8 cm, but 20 cm is optimal for the forearm. On the hand, every millimeter possible must be kept on the thumb. On the other fingers, it is necessary to consider whether a stiff and obstructing finger will be more harmful than a shorter, painless, and mobile stump. We always strive for a good tactile surface on the palmar side (Maňák, 2005).

One of the essential elements of caring for a stump is bandaging it with an elastic bandage, which contributes to shaping it into the desired shape. The bandage is tied more tightly distally and loosely proximally to prevent edema (Scott, 2017). The stump created should not be too wide or too narrow to allow a tight fitting of the prosthesis.

When evaluating the amputated stump, we note the following:

1. Resting position: the patient stands with support, the pelvis must be horizontal, and the stump must be relaxed. We note the deviation from the

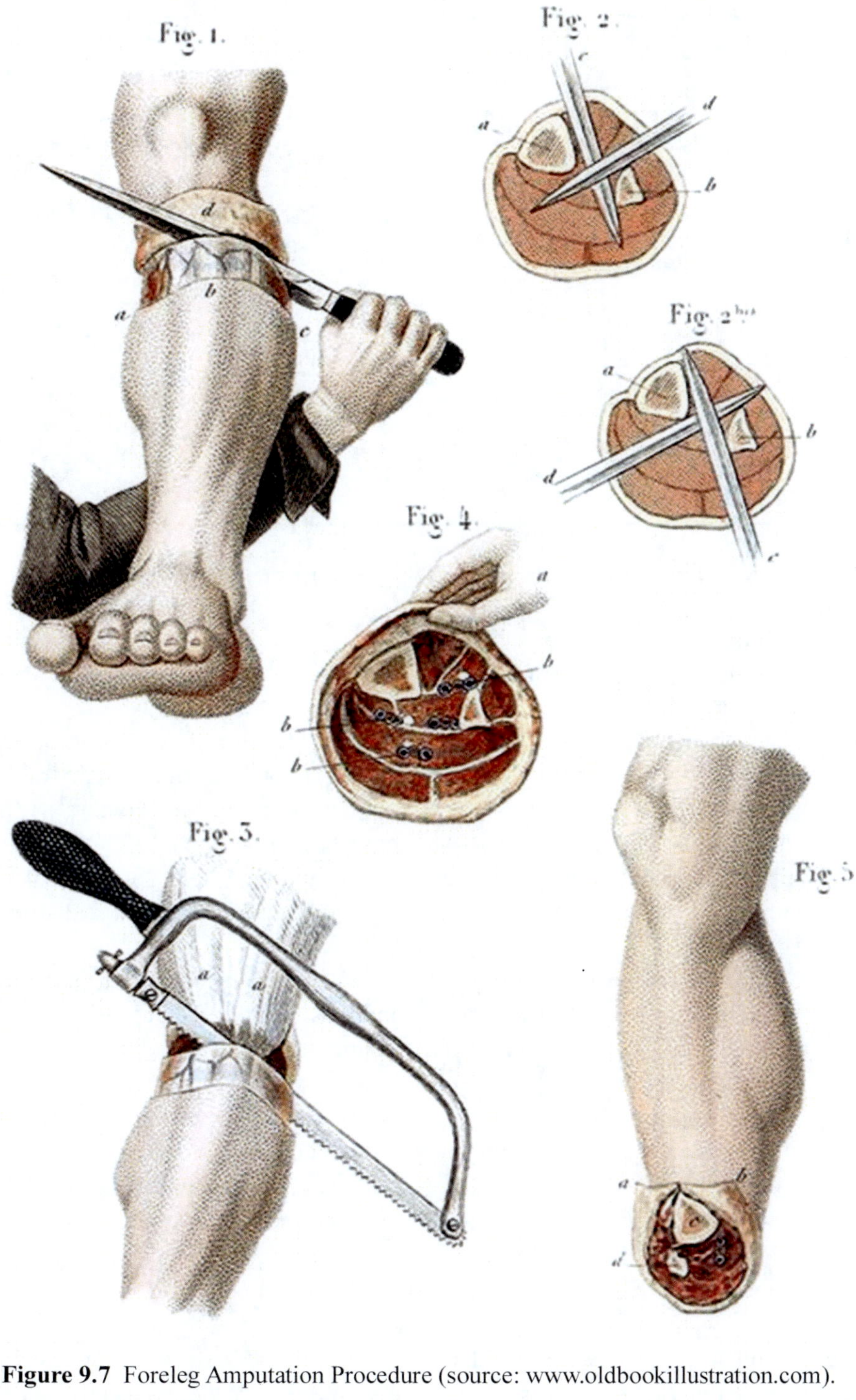

Figure 9.7 Foreleg Amputation Procedure (source: www.oldbookillustration.com).

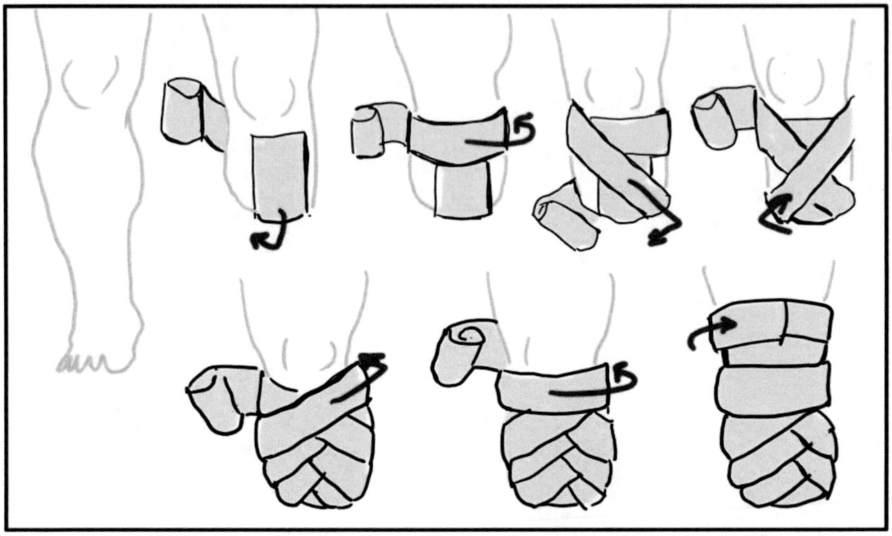

Figure 9.8 Procedure for bandaging and shaping of the stump after amputation of the lower leg (source: www.medicowesome.com).

physiological position, which is characteristic for each type of stump and level of amputation.

2. Length: the length is measured from the gap of the last preserved joint to the top of the stump. It gives us information about the functionality of the stump and the possibilities of controlling the prosthesis. Generally, the longer the stump, the easier it is to control the prosthesis.
3. Shape: depends on the type of amputation and the quality of the soft tissues of the stump. For prosthetics, a cylindrical or slightly conical stump is best.
4. Mobility: consists of the range of movement and the force that performs the given movement. We note active and passive mobility and the causes of their deviations, for example, muscle contracture or joint mobility disorder.
5. Load capacity and carrying capacity: we distinguish between load-bearing and non-load-bearing stumps. With the load-bearing stumps, it is possible to lean on the mat with part of the body weight without pain and damage to soft structures. The insufficient load-bearing capacity of the stump is mainly affected by poorly located scars, fixed scars to the base, osteophytes on the edge of the stump, bone necrosis, neuromas near the stump, etc. (Brozmanová et al. 1990, Křivánek, Eis 1972).

For wound healing, it is appropriate to use the so-called VAC (vacuum-assisted closure) therapy. It is a non-invasive treatment method, the essence of which is local negative pressure to promote wound healing and fluid drainage. In addition, it helps moisturize the healing wound, reduces bacterial contamination of the wound, and stimulates faster tissue granulation. This means the treatment time is shortened by applying negative pressure to the wound. VAC therapy is used for extensive open wounds, post-traumatic wounds, osteomyelitis, diabetic, and pressure ulcers (Fialová & Vinter, 2008). They can be used to prevent glenohumeral or elbow joint contractures. If contractures begin to develop, more intensive rehabilitation involving strengthening the muscles of the contralateral limb or using gentle passive movements and stretching may be necessary (Scott, 2017).

Complications after amputations

Local:

1. hematoma – leads to infection, necrosis, and pain; when it enlarges, revision of the stump is necessary
2. necrosis - if it is of a smaller scale, the wound can heal per secundam; if it spreads, a necrectomy is necessary
3. gangrene – begins with local ischemia and arises from an inadequate level of amputation or arterial occlusion; re-amputation at the ideal level is necessary.
4. edema – caused mainly by an inappropriate bandage, resulting in a pear-shaped stump, which is more difficult for prosthetics.
5. contracture – it is a permanent shortening of the tissue without the possibility of stretching it to a physiological position; prevention is proper rehabilitation
6. wound dehiscence - requires revision, hygiene, bandages, and resuture
7. fracture at the site of the stump
8. infection – initially necessary targeted ATB treatment, later revision with the introduction of a drain and with irrigation lavage
9. pain - also Phantom pain, caused by incorrect treatment of the stump due to nerve endings

Total:

1. psychological complication – necessary support of a psychologist and rehabilitation
2. morbidity and mortality – in polytraumas

The study by American authors aimed to examine the association between femoral amputation status and long-term risk of a major cardiac event in those who underwent amputation for either vascular or traumatic reasons. The association between using a prosthesis and a major heart attack risk was also investigated.

This observational study calculated the risk over 30 years, and the results suggest that the high risk of initial mortality resulting from amputation may prevent many amputees from developing cardiovascular disease. In their study, mortality among individuals with vascular amputation was 28% at one year and 45% at five years, which is lower than previously reported mortality ranges of 43–54% at one year and 40–90% at five years.

The frequency of perioperative cardiac events has been reported to be higher in subjects undergoing femoral amputation than those undergoing transtibial amputation - 6.8 and 3.6%, respectively.

Several studies have revealed that only about a quarter of individuals with femoral amputations receive a prosthesis. A 10-year increase in age in the civilian population resulted in a 54% reduction in the likelihood of them using a prosthesis. Similarly, a study of older American veterans revealed that a 10-year age increase reduced the possibility of receiving a prosthesis by 78%. Those who could walk independently before amputation were almost 30 times more likely to receive a prosthesis than those who could not walk independently. Interestingly, the time elapsed between surgery and the decision to have a prosthesis was associated with an increased likelihood of receiving a prosthesis during the first three months after amputation. These data illustrate the lack of consistent, reliable prosthesis prescriptions. It has not been proven that receiving a prosthesis is associated with a reduced risk of a major cardiac event after amputation.

Within the phantom limb syndrome, we distinguish between phantom pain, phantom sensations, and stump pain (pain in the residual limb). Lejčko and Skála (2002) report that, according to studies, phantom limb syndrome occurs in 60-85% of amputees, with excruciating pain occurring in 10%. Perry et al. (2018) reported that 85% of amputees experience painful sensations or phantom pain immediately after surgery or develop within days to weeks. Among these sensations are itching, pressure, or changes in the temperature sensation and the perception of a non-existent limb in space—the more proximal the amputation height, the higher the incidence of phantom limb syndrome.

Phantom pain (phantom limb pain)

According to the WHO, pain is an unpleasant sensory and emotional experience associated with direct or imminent tissue damage or described in terms of such damage. This addition applies to phantom pain, the pain in a non-existent part of the limb. Lejčko and Skála (2002) define phantom pain as pain related to a surgically or traumatically removed body part, usually in its non-existent integrity. The pain in the amputated leg is often similar to that in the limb before amputation and is mainly localized in the distal part of the missing limb. This pain is not associated with mechanical pressure on the stump (Winkelstein, 2013). Patients most often describe the pain as burning, spasmodic, cutting, stabbing, and twisting, like pricking with a needle or stabbing with a knife. They have sensations of painful pinching, crushing, and squeezing. Often the phantom limb is perceived in an unnatural, twisted position. Sometimes there are attacks of sharp, excruciating, but relatively short pain. The pain tends to recede over time; for some, it may disappear completely in 1-2 years (Lejčko and Skála, 2002). Murphy (2013) further states that phantom pain is often described as dull, burning, stabbing, electrifying, or the sensation that a non-existent limb is being torn off. Precipitating factors can include stress and cold. Phantom pain is thought to be caused by the central nervous system misjudging stimuli from the residual limb as stimuli from the missing limb. Psychological factors and the amount of blood flow to the stump can also play a role (Winkelstein, 2013). According to Tichý (2005), phantom pain could be understood as the result of the overproductive activity of cortical and subcortical structures. Cortical sensory areas that no longer receive sensory information or receive it distorted can receive replacement sensory stimuli from neighboring structures. As a result, stimuli from a non-existent limb are recorded. The sudden interruption of normal sensory activity, which is subsequently replaced by an abnormal afferent, is decisive for developing phantom pains. In general, peripheral (amputation stump and dissected peripheral nerve), central (spinal cord and brain), and psychogenic influences can be applied (Lejčko and Skála, 2002). In general, phantom pain can be treated conservatively or with surgical techniques.

Conservative treatment:

Local stump therapy uses massage techniques and soft tissue techniques to reduce muscle tension.

Application of injectable corticoids and opioids epidurally or intraspinally.

Electrostimulation of affected nerves.

Pharmacological treatment: includes the use of opioid analgesics, adjuvant analgesics (anticonvulsants, tricyclic antidepressants of the first generation), and nonsteroidal antirheumatic drugs.

Physical therapy - application of analgesic TENS currents - Transcutaneous electro neurostimulation (Varshney, 2018).

Surgical methods of treatment:

Removal and ablation of various nerve structures in the brain or spinal cord.
Ablation of a neuroma in the stump, in the case of evidence that it causes neuropathic pain; however, it is typically connected with stump pain.

Rehabilitation is essential to patient care and is necessary to achieve the desired goals. The condition after limb amputation requires a complex therapeutic approach, containing knowledge and procedures of orthopedics, orthotics, neurology, pain therapy, social and work rehabilitation, and psychology (Kolář et al., 2009). The general goal of amputation rehabilitation is to help the patient achieve the highest possible level of functionality and independence and improve the overall quality of life physically, psychologically, and socially.

The rehabilitation plan should therefore take into account the patient's age. At the same time, it can be assumed that the older the patient, the more complex and lengthy the adaptation and rehabilitation will be, and the difficulties will tend to become chronic. The patient's social background plays a vital role in the patient's daily activities. Even though there is an overall effort for the greatest possible independence of the patient, the help of the patient's family and surroundings can significantly help, especially in the initial stages after amputation. The patient's environment should not be a barrier but a facilitator. This means the patient should have factors stimulating him to work with the affected limb, improving its functionality.

References

BARČOVÁ, H., NEDVĚDOVÁ, I. Praktické využití standardu léčebné rehabilitace u pacientů po amputaci dolní končetiny ve stehně. Lékařské listy. Příloha zdravotnických novin, 2001, roč. 50, č. 29, s. 20-23.

Boucek P. Advanced diabetic neuropathy—A point of no return? Rev. Diabet. Stud. 2006;3:143–150. doi: 10.1900/RDS.2006.3.143.

Boulton A.J. Diabetic neuropathy and foot complications. Handbook Clin. Neurol. 2014;126:97–107.

Boulton A.J. The diabetic foot: Grand overview, epidemiology, and pathogenesis. Diabet./Metab. Res. Rev. 2008;24:S3–S6. doi: 10.1002/dmrr.833.

Boulton A.J. The pathway to foot ulceration in diabetes. Med. Clin. N. Am. 2013;97:775–790. doi 10.1016/j.mcna.2013.03.007.

BROZMANOVÁ, B. a kol. Ortopedická protetika. Martin: Osveta, 1990. 478 s. ISBN 80- 217-0133-1.

CAPKO, J. Základy fyziatrické léčby. Praha: Grada Publishing, 1998. 394 s. ISBN 80- 7169-341-3.

DAĎOVÁ, K. Sport osob se zdravotním postižením. In MÁČEK, M., RADVANSKÝ, J. et al. Fyziologie a klinické aspekty pohybové aktivity. Praha: Galén, 2011. s 233-237. ISBN 978-80-7262-695-3.

DOBEŠ, M. et al. Diagnostika a terapie funkčních poruch pohybového systému (manuální terapie) pro fyzioterapeuty. Horní Bludovice: Domiga, 2011. 76 s. ISBN 978-80-902222- 4-3. DRÁPELOVÁ, E. Fototerapie a Magnetoterapie. Prednášky z predmetu: Fyzikální terapie III. Brno: MU, 2013.

Dungl P. et al. Ortopedie, Grada, 2014, ISBN: 9788024743578.

DVOŘÁK, R. Základy kinezioterapie. Olomouc: Univerzita Palackého v Olomouci, 2003. 104 s. ISBN 80-244-0609-8.

EIS, E., KŘIVÁNEK, F. Ortopedie, traumatologie a ortopedická protetika. Praha: Avicenum, 1972. 382 s.

FAKULTNÍ NEMOCNICE OLOMOUC. Péče o jizvu. [cit. 12.2.2014] Dostupné na World Wide Web: http://www.fnol.cz/oddeleni-plasticke-a-esteticke-chirurgie -sluzbysekce_396.html MINISTERSTVO PRÁCE A SOCIÁLNÍCH VĚCÍ. Posudková služba. 31.12.2013 [cit. 15.2.2014] Dostupné na World Wide Web: http://www.mpsv.cz/cs/7228 43. MINISTERSTVO PRÁCE A SOCIÁLNÍCH VĚCÍ. Dávky pro osoby se zdravotním postižením. [cit. 15.2.2014] Dostupné na World Wide Web: http://www.mpsv.cz/cs/8#dsp 44.

Fialová, J. & Vinter, R. : V.A.C. Technologie vacuum assisted closure. Traumatické oddělení FN Olomouc. 2008 , Retrieved 27.3.2019 from The World Wide Web: https://www.fnol.cz/pdf/trauma/technologie.pdf.

Gilbey S.G. Neuropathy and foot problems in diabetes. Clin. Med. 2004;4:318–323. doi: 10.7861/clinmedicine.4-4-318.

GÚTH, A. et al. Vyšetrovacie metodiky v rehabilitácii pre fyzioterapeutov. Bratislava: Liečreh Gúth, 2008. 400 s. ISBN 80-88932-13-0. - 80

HADRABA, I. Ortopedická protetika - II. část. Praha: Karolinum, 2006. 106 s. ISBN 80- 246-1296-8.

HALADOVÁ, E. a kol. Léčebná tělesná výchova - cvičení. Brno: Národní centrum ošetřovatelství a nelékařských zdravotnických oborů, 2007. 135 s. ISBN 978-80-7013- 460-3. HALADOVÁ, E., NECHVÁTALOVÁ, L. Vyšetřovací metody hybného systému. Brno: Národní centrum ošetřovatelství a nelékařských zdravotnických oborů, 2005. 135 s. ISBN 80-7013-393-7.

HROMÁDKOVÁ, J. a kol. Fyzioterapie. Jinočany: H & H, 2002. 428 s. ISBN 80-86022- 45-5. 14. JANDA, V. a kol. Svalové funkční testy. Praha: Grada Publishing, 2004. 325 s. ISBN 978- 80-247-0722-5.

INTEGROVANÝ PORTÁL MPSV. Průkaz osoby se zdravotním postižením. 29.12.2011 [cit. 15.2.2014] Dostupné na World Wide Web: http://portal.mpsv.cz /soc/dzp/prukaz 45. INTEGROVANÝ PORTÁL MPSV. Pracovní rehabilitace. [cit. 15.2.2014] Dostupné na World Wide Web: https://portal.mpsv.cz/upcr/kp/ pha/pracovni_rehabilitac

JIRKOVSKÁ, A. Syndrom diabetické nohy. Praha: Maxdorf, 2006. 397 s. ISBN 80-7345- 095-X.

KLUSOŇOVÁ, E., PITNEROVÁ, J. Rehabilitační ošetřování pacientů s těžkými poruchami hybnosti. Brno: Národní centrum ošetřovatelství a nelékařských zdravotnických oborů, 2005. 117 s. ISBN 80-7013-423-2.

KOCIOVÁ, K. a kol. Základy fyzioterapie. Martin: Osveta, 2013. 238 s. ISBN 978-80- 8063-389-9.

KOLÁŘ, P. et al. Rehabilitace v klinické praxi. Praha: Galén, 2009. 713 s. ISBN 978-80- 7262-657-1.

KOZÁKOVÁ, D., JANURA, M., ROSICKÝ, J. Problematika pooperačního pahýlu u pacientů s transtibiální amputací pohledem fyzioterapeuta, biomechanika a protetika. Rehabilitace a fyzikální lékařství, 2009, roč. 16, č. 3, s. 102-108. ISSN 1211-2658. - 81

KUBEŠ, R. Amputace. In DUNGL, P. Ortopedie. Praha: Grada Publishing, 2005. s 165- 176. ISBN 80-247-0550-8

KUBÍNKOVÁ, D., KŘÍŽOVÁ A. Ergoterapie. Olomouc: Univerzita Palackého v Olomouci, 1997. 95 s. ISBN 80-7067-698-1.

LÁNIK, V., LÁNIKOVÁ, V., DUDA, E. Rehabilitácia amputovaných. Bratislava: Obzor, 1974. 79 s.

LEJČKO, J. Fantomová bolest. Lékařské listy. Příloha zdravotnických novin, 2002, roč. 51, č. 25, s. 18-20.

Lejčko J. et al.: Fantomová bolest, Lékařské listy, Príloha zdravotnických novin, 2002, roč. 51, č. 25, s.18-20.

Lobmann R. Diabetic foot syndrome. Der Internist. 2011;52:539–548. doi: 10.1007/ s00108-010-2733.

Maňák P., Wondrák E.: Traumatologie: repetitorium pro studující lékařství. Olomouc: Univerzita Palackého, Hanex Olomouc, 2005, ISBN-13: 978-80-244-1009-8.

MATĚJÍCEK, M. Ortopedická protetika. In DUNGL, P. Ortopedie. Praha: Grada Publishing, 2005. s 141-164. ISBN 80-247-0550-8.

Monteiro-Soares M., Boyko E.J., Ribeiro J., Dinis-Ribeiro L.M. Risk stratification systems for diabetic foot ulcers: A systematic review. Diabetologia. 2011;54:1190–1199. doi 10.1007/s00125-010-2030-3.

Murphy, D. P.: Fundamentals of amputation care and prosthetics, 2013, New York: Demos Medical Publishing.

PALANOVÁ, P. Amputace HKK, DKK. Cvičenie z predmetu: Léčebná rehabilitace v chirurgii, traumatologii a ortopedii. Brno: MU, 2013.

Perry, B. , Armiger, R., Wolde, M., Mcfarland, K. a., Alphonso, A. l., Monson, B. t., et al.: Clinical trial of the virtual integration environment to treat phantom limb pain with upper extremity amputation [Online], 2018, Frontiers In Neurology, 9. https://doi.org/10.3389/fneur.2018.00770

PLACHETA, Z., HRAZDIRA, L. Onemocnění a poruchy pohybového systému. In PLACHETA, Z., SIEGELOVÁ, J., ŠTEJFA, M. a spol. Zátěžová diagnostika v ambulantní a klinické praxi. Praha: Grada Publishing, 1999. s. 254-256. ISBN 80-7169- 271-9. 27. PODĚBRADSKÝ, J., PODĚBRADSKÁ, R. Fyzikální terapie: manuál a algoritmy. Praha: Grada Publishing, 2009. 200 s. ISBN 978-80-247-2899-5.

PODĚBRADSKÝ, J., VAŘEKA, I. Fyzikální terapie I. Praha: Grada Publishing, 1998. 264 s. ISBN 80-7169-661-7.

Risse A. Syndróm diabetickej nohy – interdisciplinárna výzva. Hamostaseológia. 2007; 27 :117-122.

Rumenapf G., Dittler S., Morbach S., Amendt K., Radu A. The vascular surgeon's role in interdisciplinary treatment of diabetic foot syndrome. Der Chir. Z. Fuer Alle Geb. Der Oper. Med. 2008;79:535–545.

RYBKA, J. Diabetes mellitus - komplikace a přidružená onemocnění: diagnostické a léčebné postupy. Praha: Grada Publishing, 2007. 317 s. ISBN 978-80-247-1671-8.

Said G. Diabetic neuropathy. Handbook Clin. Neurol. 2013;115:579–589

Sandireddy R., Yerra V.G., Areti A., Komirishetty P., Kumar A. Neuroinflammation and oxidative stress in diabetic neuropathy: Futuristic strategies based on these targets. Int. J. Endocrinol. 2014;2014:674987.

Scott, G.E.: Elbow and above-elbow amputations technique, 2017, Retrieved 14.3.2019 from Medscape database on the World Wide Web: https://emedicine.medscape .com/article/1237886-technique.

SIEGELOVÁ, J. a kol. Pokyny pro vypracování bakalářské práce v oboru fyzioterapie a léčebná rehabilitace. Brno: Masarykova univerzita, 2004. 17 s. ISBN 80-210-3485-8. - 82 - 31. SMUTNÝ, M. Informace pro pacienty po amputaci končetiny. Praha: Federace ortopedických protetiků technických oborů, 2009. 64 s. ISBN 978-80-254-3820-6.

Singh V.P., Bali A., Singh N., Jaggi A.S. Advanced glycation end products and diabetic complications. Korean J. Physiol. Pharmacol. 2014;18:1–14. doi: 10.4196/ kjpp.2014.18.1.1.

SOSNA, A. a kol. Základy ortopedie. Praha: Triton, 2001. 175 s. ISBN 80-7254-202-8. 33. SVOBODOVÁ, J. Prednášky z predmetu: Úvod do rehabilitace. Brno: MU, 2011. 34. VOTAVA, J. a kol. Ucelená rehabilitace osob se zdravotním postižením. Praha: Karolinum, 2003. 207 s. ISBN 80-246-0708-5.

Tichý, J.: Phantom pain. Bolest, 2005, 8(4), 203-216 [cit. 2019-01-17]. ISSN 12120634.

Van Battum P., Schaper N., Prompers L., Apelqvist J., Jude E. Differences in minor amputation rate in diabetic foot disease throughout Europe are in part explained by differences in disease severity at presentation. Diabet. Med. J. Br. Diabet. Assoc. 2011;28:199–205. doi: 10.1111/j.1464-5491.2010.03192.

Varshney, M. K. : Essential orthopedics: principles and practice, 2018, Volume 2. New Delhi: The Health Sciences Publisher.

VRABLICOVÁ, M. a kol. Komplexní rehabilitační péče u pacientů po amputaci dolní končetiny. Rehabilitace a fyzikální lékařství, 2008, roč. 15, č. 3, s. 105-109. ISSN 1211- 2658.

WAY, L. a kol. Současná chirurgická diagnostika a léčba. 2. díl. Praha: Grada Publishing, 1998. s. 807-1659. ISBN 80-7169-397-9.

Winkelstein, B. A.: Orthopaedic biomechanics, 2013, Boca Raton: CRC Press.

ZEMAN, M. et al. Speciální chirurgie. Praha: Galén, 2004. 575 s. ISBN 80-7262-260-9. Internetové zdroje: ÚSTAV ZDRAVOTNICKÝCH INFORMACÍ A STATISTIKY ČR. Péče o nemocné cukrovkou 2012. 2012 [cit. 4.1.2014] Dostupné na World Wide Web: http://www.uzis.cz/katalog/zdravotnicka -statistika/pece-nemocne-cukrovkou 39. MROČKOVÁ, I. Rehabilitace po amputacích pro diabetické komplikace. Sestra, 2011, č. 6 [cit. 6.2.2014] Dostupné na World Wide Web: http://zdravi.e15.cz/clanek/sestra/rehabilitace -po-amputacich-pro-diabeticke-komplikace460359 40. M. A. ORTOPEDICKÁ PROTETIKA s.r.o. Rady a návody pro pacienty. [cit. 9.2.2014] Dostupné na World Wide Web: http://maprotetika.cz/navod.html - 83 - 41.

Zenker J., Ziegler D., Chrast R. Novel pathogenic pathways in diabetic neuropathy. Trends Neurosci. 2013;36:439–449. doi: 10.1016/j.tins.2013.04.008.

Ziegler D., Keller J., Maier C., Pannek J. Diabetic neuropathy. Exp. Clin. Endocrinol. Diabet. Off. J. Ger. Soc. Endocrinol. Ger. Diabet. Assoc. 2014;122:406–415. doi: 10.1055/s-0034-1366435.

Zimmermann A., Reeps C., Hartl F., Ockert S., Eckstein H.H. The diabetic foot. Der Chir. Z. Fuer Alle Geb. Der Oper. Med. 2009;80:430–436.

Chapter 10

Podiatric Care

Peter Zavacký, MD*
Department of Surgery, Faculty of Medicine, Pavol Jozef Šafárik University in Košice and University Hospital, Košice, Slovakia

Abstract

Podiatry is a medical field that deals with studying, diagnosing, treating, and preventing diseases of the foot, ankle, associated tissues, and structures by all appropriate methods. Multidisciplinary cooperation is necessary to treat and prevent diabetic foot syndrome successfully. Follow-up of patients with diabetic foot syndrome by experienced professionals and interdisciplinary collaboration can help reduce severe consequences, including amputation and cardiovascular mortality. Increasing evidence promotes the use of podiatry services within the community to facilitate the care of diabetic foot, with the latest evidence showing a reduction in hospitalizations and preventable amputations. In addition, patient education has also been shown to be an essential element in delaying the onset or recurrence of diabetic foot ulcers.

Key Words: podiatry, diabetic foot, ulcer, infection, hyperkeratosis

Podiatry is a medical field that deals with the study, diagnosis, treatment, and prevention of diseases of the foot, ankle, associated tissues, and structures using all appropriate methods, as well as the local manifestation of overall processes in this area. Medical care for high-risk patients is also essential. It is necessary to define that the foot is the part of the lower limb distal to the ankle (talocrural) joint, and the primary domain of the field is the treatment of diabetic foot syndrome. According to the latest edition of the International Consensus, diabetic

---

* Corresponding Author's Email: peterzavacky963@gmail.com

In: Diabetic Foot
Editor: Martina Zavacká
ISBN: 979-8-89113-019-7

foot is defined as infection, ulceration, or tissue destruction of the foot associated with neuropathy and/or peripheral artery disease in the lower extremities of people with diabetes. Successful treatment and prevention of diabetic foot syndrome depend on a holistic approach – it is seen as part of multi-organ involvement. Therefore, the teamwork of several experts is necessary. The key role in this team is played mainly by an internist with a diabetologist, an angiologist, a vascular surgeon, and a surgeon with podiatric training. They manage diabetes control, prevent and treat comorbidities, cooperate in diagnosing malnutrition and nutritional therapy, and the early diagnosis and effective treatment of infections. Last but not least, in cooperation with other experts, the internist works on treating the lower limb ischemia, appropriately selecting ulcer treatment and local therapy, and preventing ulcers. The main problem in podiatry is recurrent ulceration. They occur in 40% of patients in the first year after recovery. Monitoring patients with diabetic foot syndrome by experienced professionals and interdisciplinary collaboration can help reduce serious outcomes, including amputation and cardiovascular mortality. Based on the determination of the degree of risk of ulceration, they try to determine the number of control examinations of the legs and educate at-risk patients and their family members, especially regarding the local treatment of ulcerations, infections, and osteoarthropathy. The most important thing is the preventive treatment of the feet: hyperkeratosis, deformities, dry skin, and mycosis. Early and correct prevention and treatment of infection and ulceration, especially in patients with limb ischemia, significantly reduces the incidence of amputations.

The prevention and management of diabetic foot ulceration require comprehensive, well-coordinated multidisciplinary care in all healthcare facilities, as recommended by the National Institute of Health and Care Excellence (NICE) and the National Framework 'Putting Feet First.' This care modality is structured to include a 'Foot Protection Team (FPT)' working in the community, consisting of health professionals, often podiatrists, with specialist expertise in assessing and managing the diabetic foot. The FPT works closely with the 'Multidisciplinary Foot Care Team (MDFT),' which deals with diabetic foot problems in hospitals and more complex cases in the community.

Regular assessment of vascular status using FPT is of utmost importance in managing the diabetic foot to detect the presence of peripheral arterial disease (PAD). PAD is the leading risk factor for the development of ulceration, amputation, and overall mortality. Detection of PAD on a non-ulcerated leg allows for correctly identifying a risk condition and preventing ulcers. In addition, it provides a significant opportunity to modify cardiovascular risk factors that may positively affect mortality. Furthermore, fast and accurate detection of PAD in the ulcerated leg is even more critical because the time to revascularization determines ulcer healing and limb salvage. With a late diagnosis of PAD, consideration of revascularization is delayed and often inappropriate because of tissue loss or infection progression. Delayed vascular assessment and intervention reported in the literature negatively affect patient results.

Time to revascularization is potentially influenced by several variables, including factors related to the patient (e.g., delay in follow-up), the health care provider (e.g., delay in diagnosis, lack of knowledge and training), and the health care system (e.g., referral methods, waiting lists, staff). Current national datasets from England provide very little information on PAD diagnostic procedures, decision-making after suspected PAD, and the status of vascular surgery referral pathways. In this national survey of podiatry practice in the United Kingdom (UK), we aimed to examine current practices in diagnosing PAD in diabetes, decision-making when PAD is suspected, and limitations of referral pathways. This can help identify potential targets for further investigation and quality improvement.

Examination of the patient

The examination of a diabetic patient's feet begins with simply taking off the shoes, at least once a year, and in the case of high-risk patients, more often during each visit.

From the point of view of anamnesis, we first ask about difficulties, discomfort, and pain (at rest or during exertion) and locate it more closely in terms of intensity, duration, triggering moments, and symmetry (asymmetry). It is necessary to realize that diabetic patients do not have claudication pain even with significant limb ischemia. We localize and identify pathological findings on the legs: bruises, ulcerations, necrosis, infections, swelling, deformities, and their provoking factors, e.g., long walks, unsuitable shoes, increased physical exertion, temperature effects, walking barefoot. We also focus on treating diabetes, the underlying disease, and associated diseases. We are also interested in family and social anamnesis.

Physical examination

During the inspection, we observe a change in the color of the legs, pathological findings on the skin, rashes, excoriations, deformities, and edema. We also note the quality of the skin, dryness, and possible peeling, which is common with neuropathies. With motor neuropathy, muscle mass decreases, and with autonomic neuropathy, dry skin and dilated veins on the dorsum of the leg are present. With ischemia, the skin can have a wide range of coloration:

from dark red and livid to pale and bloodless. The skin is usually thin, shiny, and tense, with subcutaneous tissue atrophy. There is often a claw-like position of the toes; it is a fixed flexion position of the toes, which subsequently causes the formation of calluses on the toe pads, often leading to ulceration. A great risk of dorsal ulceration is the so-called hammer toe, where flexion deformity of the proximal interphalangeal joint is present with hyperextension of the distal interphalangeal joint. Another common deformity is hallux valgus with lateral deviation of the big toe and medial prominence of the edge of the foot. There is usually the most vulnerable place on the leg where a bruise and an ulcer are formed, especially when wearing inappropriate shoes. In hallux rigidus, there is a loss of dorsiflexion of the big toe, which leads to great pressure on the plantar area of the first toe with the formation of a callus. In Charcot osteoarthropathy, a collapsed arch can be seen with a prominence on the planta pedis and a predilection site for the formation of bruises and ulcerations. Deformities also occur after injuries, surgical procedures, collapses of the transverse arch, and atrophy of fat pads in the metatarsophalangeal area. In motor neuropathy, this arch is usually too high (pes cavus). Nails are also often deformed, which should be consulted with a dermatologist. A predisposing factor for an open wound is swelling, which impairs healing because it makes shoes uncomfortable. Bilateral edema is usually a heart and kidney failure or venous insufficiency symptom. The so-called neuropathic edema is a consequence of sympathetic denervation. It occurs due to increased blood flow to the affected limb due to massive vasodilatation caused by sympathetic denervation. Arteriovenous junctions open. Unilateral swelling is usually associated with a local pathological process. It is often an infection with erythema, gout, trauma, deep vein thrombosis, lymphedema, Charcot leg, hematoma, and pus. Loss of skin integrity covering the foot and ankle joint area is synonymous with "diabetic foot syndrome." It is also necessary to inspect the spaces between the toes. They are not always visible immediately; they can be masked by exudate, callus, nail, swelling, and redness. The infection is manifested by swelling, redness, and often purulent discharge from the wound; the surrounding skin is warm and painful, and the patient may also have a higher body temperature. Any loss of skin integrity is a gateway to infection. Necrosis is the presence of devitalized tissue - dark to black.

By palpation, we check the skin's temperature, dryness, or tension on the legs; we palpate the peripheral arteries: dorsal pedis artery, posterior tibial artery, and upward, the popliteal and femoral artery. Ischemia is manifested by loss of pulsation, coldness, and discoloration. The podiatrist should also focus on the type and quality of the patient's shoes.

Neuropathy screening

We investigate neuropathy using tendon-periosteal reflexes and qualitative and quantitative sensory reflexes. We induce reflexes with a neurological hammer, sensitivity with cotton wool, and pressure sensations with monofilament. We examine pain sensitivity with a sharp object, vibrational sensitivity with a tuning fork, thermal sensitivity with warm and cold water, and disturbance of vibrational sensitivity with a biothesiometer. An electrical conductivity test is also an option. Considering the great importance of diabetic neuropathy in anamnesis, we investigate the Neuropathy Symptom Score (NSS) and Neuropathy Disability Score (NDS). Both legs are evaluated, and at the same time, we investigate the ABI index (ankle-brachial index).

Angiopathy examination is performed as follows: Doppler measurement, ankle-brachial index (ABI), values from 0.9-1.2 are considered normal, 0.7-0.9 – mild obstruction, 0.6-0.69 – moderate obstruction, and values lower than 0.6 – severe obstruction. In critical ischemia, the ABI is lower than 0.5. Mainly in patients with mediocalcinosis, we measure ankle and toe pressures.

The International Working Group on the Diabetic Foot (IWGDF) guidelines recommend using the ABPI measurement to evaluate the diabetic foot. They recommend considering ABPI measurements less than 0.9 as abnormal and those between 0.9–1.3 as predominantly excluding PAD. Although it is generally accepted that low values (< 0.9) help detect arterial disease, evidence suggests that high values (0.9–1.3 or > 1.3) cannot reliably rule out PAD in diabetes. This is because measurements may be falsely elevated due to the presence of incompressible calcified vessels in the process of mediocalcinosis [29]. Podiatrists in the UK have shown poor knowledge of ABPI interpretation in surveys, with 44.3% either incorrectly thinking that ABPI is a reliable method for ruling out PAD in diabetes. They also showed poor knowledge of

Table 10.1 Degrees of diabetic neuropathy (Department of Vascular Surgery VUSCH)

1st degree	Subclinical peripheral sensory-motor neuropathy
2nd degree	Clinical peripheral sensory-motor neuropathy
	• a chronic painful form • an acute painful form • painless form
3rd degree	Complications of diabetic neuropathy
	• ulcerations on the skin of the leg • Charcot neuroosteoarthropathy • limb amputation

the utility of the ABPI, with only 26% of respondents routinely performing it in clinical practice. These results suggest that the IWGDF guidelines must be revised to clarify this issue.

Neuropathy may mask symptoms such as claudication and pain at rest, while arterial calcification prevents palpation of the leg pulse. Pulse palpation is also limited by variability among examiners. Great importance is also attached to assessing the audible signal of the artery using a hand-held Doppler. However, it has low sensitivity (43%) in patients with diabetes and poor diagnostic reliability.

Due to limited data and the low methodological quality of studies, there is currently little evidence to support using only one non-invasive diagnostic modality. However, limited evidence suggests that TBPI and TcPO 2 may be more demonstrative than ABPI measurements in diabetes patients. However, in the UK respondent pool, they were rarely used in clinical practice (6.2 and 0.8%), and they were also rated as the least important in clinical decision-making. The result of the survey thus indicates that there is insufficient use of TBPI and TcPO 2 within the complete assessment of PAD.

Assessment of arterial disease in diabetes

Current recommendations for podiatrists list history, pulse palpation with/without audible assessment of the Doppler wave, and ABPI as part of the standard assessment of arterial insufficiency. This is supported by the International Working Group on the Diabetic Foot (IWGDF) guidelines, which recommend a combination of history and pulse palpation in patients without active foot ulceration and the additional use of ABPI and assessment of arterial waveforms in patients with ulceration. Most survey respondents (96%) reported using a minimal combination of history and pulse palpation to evaluate for PAD. Although 86% reported using at least one additional non-invasive test (most commonly audible assessment), very few used the whole combination of history, pulse palpation, Doppler waveform assessment, and ABPI (18.8%). We also found significant differences in what varieties of tests were used across regions of the UK.

Vascular referral pathways

After PAD is suspected, it must be decided whether sending the patient for further vascular examination is appropriate. The IWGDF recommended that additional vascular imaging and revascularization be considered in patients with a leg ulcer and critical limb ischemia (toe pressure < 30 mmHg, TcPO 2 < 25 mmHg) and also in patients with a non-healing leg ulcer and evidence of PAD (ankle pressure < 50 mmHg or ABPI < 0.5). They also recommended considering vascular imaging and subsequent vascular intervention, regardless of bedside test results, when an ulcer does not heal within six weeks despite optimal management.

In a survey, up to 60% of respondents said they would refer any patient with suspected PAD and diabetes for further vascular evaluation, regardless of the ulcer status. Routine referral of patients with suspected PAD but without evidence of tissue loss is not recommended in current guidelines and increases the demand for vascular investigations. In the presence of PAD, 16.8% of respondents said that after six weeks of conservative treatment, they would only refer patients with non-healing ulcers for further evaluation, which could lead to a significant delay in treatment. Many respondents also stated that they would not request further vascular evaluation before local debridement in cases of suspected PAD. This procedure can be risky because debridement of the ischemic leg may not heal at all.

These results highlight the need for better collaboration between vascular and podiatry professionals to clarify guidelines at the local level and ensure that all healthcare providers are aware of them.

Our results indicate that podiatrists seeing more patients are more likely to have access to a vascular specialist, suggesting that this problem primarily affects those with fewer patients. The open-ended responses of podiatrists in this survey indicate that the lack of vascular specialists may be a potential barrier that requires further investigation.

After making a referral for a specialist vascular examination, nearly 70% of podiatrists reported that their patients waited longer than two weeks, with the majority waiting longer than four weeks. Long delays, lack of capacity, and too few clinical workplaces were often reported as the main limitations of vascular medicine. In the open-ended responses, some podiatrists clarified that finding and describing ulcerations significantly increased the speed of examination by a specialist. However, others noted that this was different.

Another important survey finding is the commonly perceived difficulty with the referral process for further examinations. There is some frustration with not being able to refer patients directly to vascular clinics. Most podiatrists have to make a referral through the patient's GP, which can be another source of delay. Surprisingly, more than 70% of respondents said they do not receive regular feedback on the results of vascular consultations. This is reflected in the number of people who pointed to poor communication as a limitation of special vascular examinations. This may also be because referrals are initiated through the general practitioner, who then receives the test results. It points to the need for better cooperation between vascular and podiatry workers and the improvement of established recommendations.

This survey also pointed to a lack of compliance with guidelines for detecting arterial disease in diabetes, low usage of non-invasive tests such as ABPI, TBPI, and TCO 2, and poor knowledge of ABPI interpretation among UK podiatrists. In addition, the research pointed out insufficient access to vascular specialists in Britain, particularly among podiatrists who see a lower volume of patients and cannot sufficiently make direct referrals for further vascular assessment. They have insufficient feedback regarding the evaluation of vascular outcomes and long waiting times for vascular inspection and DUS imaging. The above findings are important targets for further investigation and quality improvement.

On the patient's hands, we also examine the phenomenon of limited joint mobility - diabetic cheiroarthropathy. The patient should clasp his hands as if praying or place his hands on the mat, which these patients usually cannot do. This disorder is also present in the legs.

Assessment of the risk of diabetic foot syndrome

We pay increased attention to diabetic patients with a poor lifestyle and inadequate compensation, smokers, alcoholics, people from lower social classes, and new type 2 diabetes.

Increased self-monitoring and self-help are recommended to patients when a risk foot is detected. Daily inspection of the feet, suitable footwear, proper and frequent feet hygiene, regular and appropriate nail trimming,

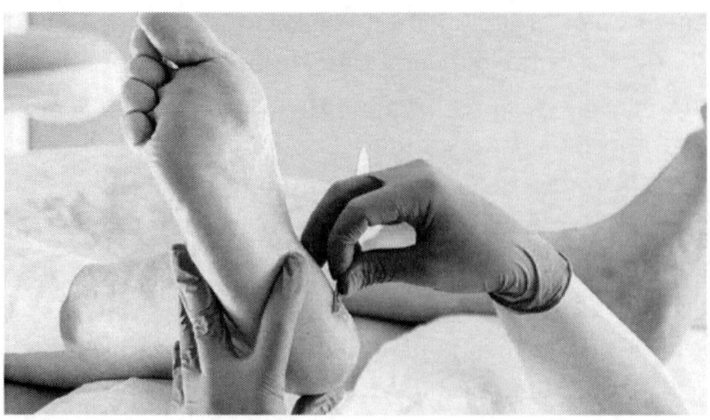

Figure 10.1 Podiatric care of the diabetic foot (source: Department of Vascular Surgery VUSCH).

gentle removal of hyperkeratosis, and seeing a specialist in case of changes. In the case of neuropathy, the patient should not walk barefoot; it is necessary to deal with foot deformities, have the water temperature or the surrounding bodies checked by another person due to the risk of burns, and lubricate dry skin. Check the shoes, get used to the new shoes sufficiently, and do not expose one's feet to the sun (since the skin is dry already!).

The most common cause of ulcers is wearing inappropriate shoes. The suitable preventive shoe should have a stiff, rigid sole to reduce pressure on the foot and a flexible and high, flat footbed. The surest fixation is lacing. It must be of sufficient length and width so the toes have enough room to move sideways and upwards. Shoes should be breathable, preferably leather, with a low heel. It is also necessary to feel the inside of the shoes so that there is no foreign body or that the inner lining is not destroyed. Hyperkeratosis occurs in the place of increased pressure when wearing uncomfortable shoes, especially during prolonged walking. Hyperkeratosis often covers the ulceration site, which is hemorrhagic on the surface. The skin presses on the surface, and the area is ischemic. Hyperkeratosis prevents wound healing. Therefore, its removal significantly helps the healing of ulcers and wound healing. The podiatrist removes it with a scalpel while saving healthy skin in the vicinity - sharp debridement. On larger surfaces, it can be removed with a sander or pumice stone (preferably after a bath), smoothened with a file, and greased with petroleum jelly. The skin can be removed non-surgically by the patient. The patient should cut the nails straight, preferably after a bath. It is advisable to lighten the place of ulceration, e.g., with a dynamic insole adapted to the foot's shape, the so-called 'half shoes,' 'walker' orthosis, or a special fixation cast. Do not forget about local antiseptics, which, although they interfere with the spontaneous healing of the wound, disinfect the area and prevent the penetration and spread of infection.

Table 10.2 Levels of the risk of ulceration with the frequency of check-ups Department of Vascular Surgery VUSCH

Risk degree	Clinical picture	Frequency of check-ups
0	No neuropathy, no ischemia	Once a year
1	Neuropathy present	Once every six months
2	Present neuropathy and ischemia with/or without leg deformities	Once in 3 months
3	History of ulcerations	On every visit

Other treatment procedures in the future may be hyperbaric oxygen therapy, negative pressure treatment, or stem cell treatment, which are all still in the experimental stage.

Podiatric clinics

There are few of these specialized workplaces in Slovakia. Their task is primarily identifying at-risk patients, educating patients and their family members, examining and treating wounds, long-term follow-up of open wounds and their treatment progression, and solving urgent problems on the feet of people with diabetes. Cooperation with a diabetologist, angiologist, neurologist, surgeon, angiosurgeon, dermatologist, orthopedist, prosthetist, physiotherapist, podiatrist, radiologist, or other specialists is necessary and self-evident. A study by British authors Gibson et al. from 2014 demonstrated that diabetic foot care by a pedicurist was associated with a lower risk of lower limb amputation and a reduced hospitalization rate.

According to international guidelines, diabetic foot care should be organized in three degrees:

Degree 1: minimal model, foot examination, problem detection, risk group screening, preventive treatment, patient education, focusing on choosing the proper footwear, and preventing foot trauma. The medical team comprises a doctor, a nurse, and a podiatrist.

Degree 2: intermediate podiatric clinic model already treats and solves infection and self-management of ulceration and infection. The team consists of a diabetologist, a surgeon, a nurse, a podiatrist, and a prosthetist. It is usually located in a hospital.

Degree 3: center for the diabetic foot, where experts in the given issue already come together: a diabetologist and a surgeon are an inherent part, a physiotherapist, a microbiologist, a dermatologist, a psychiatrist, a plaster technician, a prosthetist, a podiatrist, a nurse, and educators are also available.

In the 1980s, vascular surgeons David Campbell, Gary Gibbons, and Frank Pomposelli joined the group of Dr. Wheelock, where they started an annual conference on the diabetic foot in 1981, with podiatrists as faculty members. This conference generated national interest and played an essential role in advancing the concept of a multidisciplinary team approach to improving the care of the diabetic foot. Podiatrists participated as team members. This relationship developed into a successful long-term partnership between vascular surgeons and podiatrists and served as a model for creating other teams across the United States.

Principles of management of diabetic foot syndrome

Management is multidisciplinary, primarily to prevent the onset and progression of the disease. The basis is to care for the wound, keep it free of microbial superinfection, relieve pressure on the affected part of the leg, ensure good blood circulation, and compensate for the underlying disease.

Good wound healing can be ensured if:

- we reduce ischemia (revascularization of the limb)
- we reduce edema
- we relieve (remove) the pressure on the open wound
- we treat the infection
- we provide regular debridement

From the point of view of an open wound, the following are important: location, size, base, edges, depth of the wound, presence of infection, and ischemia.

For simple and more profound but localized wounds, debridement can also be done at the podiatric clinic. For deeper, heavily infected wounds, surgical intervention is required.

Cost-effective management should focus not only on short-term costs until healing but also on long-term costs since leg ulcers and amputation, in particular, are associated with an increased incidence of re-ulceration and lifelong disability. A multidisciplinary approach, including a prevention strategy, patient and staff education, and multifactorial treatment of leg ulcers, has been reported to reduce amputation rates (by more than 50%), rehabilitation, and the need for home care and social services for disabled patients. Therefore, one of the most important steps to reduce the cost of treating a diabetic foot is to avoid amputations.

The primary therapy in the intervention of diabetic complications of the lower limbs is prevention. Increasing evidence supports the use of podiatry services within the community to facilitate diabetic foot care. The most recent evidence shows a reduction in preventable hospitalizations and amputations. In addition, patient education has also been shown to be an essential element in delaying the onset or recurrence of diabetic foot ulcers. This includes providing information on essential foot care advice, including advice on appropriate footwear and wound care. A survey conducted to evaluate the effectiveness of patient education on diabetic foot care demonstrated a positive impact on patients' health beliefs, as evidenced by a statistically significant positive change in weight.

References

Adam DJ, Beard JD, Cleveland T, Bell J, Bradbury AW, Forbes JF, et al. Bypass versus angioplasty in severe ischemia of the leg (BASIL): a multicentre, randomized controlled trial. Lancet. 2005;366(9501):1925–1934. doi: 10.1016/S0140-6736(05)67704-5.

Alavi A, Sibbald RG, Nabavizadeh R, Valaei F, Coutts P, Mayer D. Audible handheld Doppler ultrasound determines reliable and inexpensive exclusion of significant peripheral arterial disease. Vascular. 2015;23(6):622–629. doi 10.1177/1708538114568703. [PubMed]

Apelqvist J, Elgzyri T, Larsson J, Löndahl M, Nyberg P, Thörne J. Factors related to the outcome of neuroischemic/ischemic foot ulcer in diabetic patients. J Vasc Surg. 2011;53(6):1582–1588.e2. doi: 10.1016/j.jvs.2011.02.006.

Apelqvist J, Larsson J, Agardh CD. The importance of peripheral pulses, peripheral edema, and local pain for the outcome of diabetic foot ulcers. Diabet Med. 1990;7(7):590–594. doi 10.1111/j.1464-5491.1990.tb01454.

Apelqvist J, Larsson J. What is the most effective way to reduce the incidence of amputation in the diabetic foot? Diabetes Metab Res Rev. 2000;16(Suppl1): S75–S83. doi: 10.1002/1520-7560(200009/10)16:1+<::AID-DMRR139>3.0.CO;2-8.

Apelqvist JAP, Lepäntalo MJA. The ulcerated leg: when to revascularize. Diabetes Metab Res Rev. 2012;28:30–35. doi: 10.1002/dmrr.2259.

Armstrong DG, Kanda VA, Lavery LA, Marston W, Mills JL, Boulton AJM. Mind the gap: disparity between research funding and costs of Care for Diabetic Foot Ulcers. Diabetes Care. 2013;36(7)

Boyko EJ, Ahroni JH, Davignon D, Stensel V, Prigeon RL, Smith DG. Diagnostic utility of the history and physical examination for peripheral vascular disease among patients with diabetes mellitus. J Clin Epidemiol. 1997;50(6):659–668. doi: 10.1016/S0895-4356(97)00005

Brownrigg JRW, Hinchliffe RJ, Apelqvist J, Boyko EJ, Fitridge R, Mills JL, et al. Effectiveness of bedside investigations to diagnose peripheral artery disease among people with diabetes mellitus: a systematic review. Diabetes Metab Res Rev. 2016;32(Suppl 1):119–127. doi: 10.1002/dmrr.2703.

Brownrigg JRW, Schaper NC, Hinchliffe RJ. Diagnosis and assessment of peripheral arterial disease in the diabetic foot. Diabet Med. 2015;32:738–747. doi: 10.1111/dme.12749.

Diabetes UK. Fixing footcare in Sheffield: Improving the pathway. 2015. Available from: https://diabetes-resources-production.s3-eu-west-1.amazonaws.com/diabetes-storage/2017-08/Footcare%20Case%20Study%201-%20Improving%20the%20pathway%20in%20Sheffield%20%28February%202015%29.pdf. Accessed 23 Feb 2017.

DiabetesUK . Putting feet first: national minimum skills Framework. 2011.

Elgzyri T, Larsson J, Nyberg P, Thörne J, Eriksson K-F, Apelqvist J. Early revascularization after admittance to a diabetic foot center affects the healing probability of ischemic foot ulcer in patients with diabetes. Eur J Vasc Endovasc Surg. 2014;48(4):440–446. doi: 10.1016/j.ejvs.2014.06.041.

Elo S, Kyngäs H. The qualitative content analysis process. J Adv Nurs Blackwell Publishing Ltd. 2008;62(1):107–115.

Forsythe RO, Hinchliffe RJ. Assessment of foot perfusion in patients with a diabetic foot ulcer. Diabetes Metab Res Rev. 2016;32:232–238. doi: 10.1002/dmrr.275

Gibson TB, Driver VR, Wrobel JS, Christina JR, Bagalman E, DeFrancis R, et al. Podiatrist care and outcomes for patients with diabetes and foot ulcer. Int Wound J 2014; 11: 641–648.

Health and Social Care Information Centre. NHS Workforce Statistics - July 2016, provisional statistics: staff Group, Area, and Level. Available from: https://digital.nhs.uk/media/29698/NHS-Workforce-Statistics-July-2016-Provisional-Statistics-Staff-Group-Area-and-Level-/Any/nhs-work-stat-july-2016-area-levl. Accessed 15 Mar 2018.

Health and Social Care Information Centre. NHS Workforce Statistics - July 2016, Provisional statistics: CSV tables. Available from: https://digital.nhs.uk/media/29700/NHS-Workforce-Statistics-July-2016-Provisional-Statistics-CSV-tables/Any/nhs-work-stat-july-2016-csv. Accessed 15 Mar 2018.

Hinchliffe RJ, Brownrigg JRW, Apelqvist J, Boyko EJ, Fitridge R, Mills JL, et al. IWGDF guidance on the diagnosis, prognosis, and management of peripheral artery disease in patients with foot ulcers in diabetes. Diabetes Metab Res Rev. 2016;32(Suppl 1):37–44. doi: 10.1002/dmrr.2698.

Leese GP, Stang D. Kedy a ako vykonať audit služby diabetickej nohy. Diabetes Metab Res Rev. 2016; 32 :311-317. doi: 10.1002/dmrr.2749.

Lundin M, Wiksten JP, Peräkylä T, Lindfors O, Savolainen H, Skyttä J, et al. Distal pulse palpation: is it reliable? World J Surg. 1999;23(3):252–255. doi: 10.1007/PL00013177.

Mills JL, Beckett WC, Taylor SM. The diabetic foot: consequences of delayed treatment and referral. South Med J. 1991;84(8):970–974. doi 10.1097/00007611-199108000-00009.

National Diabetes Foot Care Audit Report 2014–2015. Available from: https://www.hqip.org.uk/resource/national-diabetes-foot-care-audit-report-2014-2015/. Accessed 23 Feb 2017.

National Institute for Health and Care Excellence (NICE). Diabetic foot problems: prevention and management (NICE guideline; NG 19). August 2015. https://www.nice.org.uk/guidance/ng19. Accessed 23 Feb 2017.

NHSScotland. NHSScotland Workforce Information Quarterly update of Staff in Post and Vacancies on 30 September 2016. Available from: https://www.isdscotland.org/Health-Topics/Workforce/Publications/2016-12-06/2016-12-06-Workforce-Report.pdf?58260744811. Accessed 15 Mar 2018.

Noronen K, Saarinen E, Albäck A, Venermo M. Analysis of the elective treatment process for critical limb Ischaemia with tissue loss: diabetic patients require rapid revascularization. Eur J Vasc Endovasc Surg. 2017;53(2):206–213. doi: 10.1016/j.ejvs.2016.10.023.

Northern Ireland Statistics and Research Agency (NISRA). Northern Ireland health and social care (HSC) workforce census March 2005 to March 2016, Department of Health. Available from: https://www.health-ni.gov.uk/sites/default/files/publications/health/hscwc-march-2016-tables.xlsx. Accessed 15 Mar 2018.

Peripheral Arterial Disease in People With Diabetes. Diabetes Care. 2003;26(12):3333 LP–341.

Prompers L, Huijberts M, Apelqvist J, Jude E, Piaggesi A, Bakker K, et al. Delivery of care to diabetic patients with foot ulcers in daily practice: results of the Eurodiale study, a prospective cohort study. Diabet Med. 2008;25(6):700–707. doi: 10.1111/j.1464-5491.2008.02445

Prompers L, Schaper N, Apelqvist J, Edmonds M, Jude E, Mauricio D, et al. Prediction of outcome in individuals with diabetic foot ulcers: focus on the differences between individuals with and without the peripheral arterial disease. The EURODIALE study. Diabetologia. Springer. 2008;51(5):747–755. Doi: 10.1007/s00125-008-0940-0.

StatsWales. Non-medical NHS staff by grade and staff Group 2016 Available from: https://statswales.gov.wales/Catalogue/Health-and-Social-Care/NHS-Staff/Non-Medical-Staff/nonmedicalnhsstaff-bystaffgroup-grade-year. Accessed 15 Mar 2018.

Tehan PE, Chuter VH. Use of hand-held Doppler ultrasound examination by podiatrists: a reliability study. J Foot Ankle Res. 2015;8:36. doi: 10.1186/s13047-015-0097-2.

Winocour PH, Morgan J, Ainsworth A, Williams DRR. Association of British Clinical Diabetologists. Association of British Clinical Diabetologists (ABCD): a survey of specialist diabetes care services in the UK, 2000. 3. Podiatry services and related foot care issues. Diabet Med. 2002;19(Suppl 4):32–38. doi: 10.1046/j.1464-5491.19.s4.8

Young MJ, McCardle JE, Randall LE, Barclay JI. Improved survival of diabetic foot ulcer patients 1995-2008: possible impact of aggressive cardiovascular risk management. Diabetes Care American Diabetes Association; 2008;31(11):2143–2147.

Chapter 11

Diabetic Polyneuropathy

Jana Pobehová, MD*
Department of Vascular Surgery, East Slovak Institute of Cardiovascular Diseases, Košice, Slovakia

Abstract

Neuropathy is a disorder of nerve function and/or its organic damage. It occurs in almost 50% of patients with diabetes and affects both somatic and autonomic nerve fibers. The process is chronic and progressive, lasting years. It is associated with diabetic retinopathy and nephropathy. The decisive treatment is long-term strict glycemic control. An acute polyneuropathy is a rare form. The chronic form is more common. The incidence is reported to be 7-20%, twice higher in type 2 diabetes, with a 50% predominance of women. Distal symmetric sensorimotor neuropathy and ischemia are decisive risk factors for developing diabetic foot syndrome.

Key Words: neuropathy, diabetes mellitus, glycemia, nerve fibers, diabetic foot syndrome

The term "neuropathy" refers to a disorder of nerve function and/or its organic damage. A simple general definition refers to diabetic neuropathy as the presence of subjective and/or objective symptoms of peripheral nerve dysfunction in patients with diabetes mellitus after excluding other causes. Neuropathy occurs in almost 50% of diabetics and affects both somatic and autonomic nerve fibers. Neuropathy plays a decisive role in the development of diabetic foot syndrome. According to the latest knowledge, patients with diabetes also include patients with prediabetes, in whom symptoms of sensitive neuropathy also appear in up

---

* Corresponding Author's Email: jana.pastvova@post.cz

In: Diabetic Foot
Editor: Martina Zavacká
ISBN: 979-8-89113-019-7

to 11% of cases. The primary task of a diabetologist is the first contact, screening, diagnosis of neuropathy, and follow-up. In preventing and treating diabetic foot, the range of specialists is expanded to include an angiologist, dermatologist, angiosurgeon, podiatrist, physiatrist, and rehabilitation workers.

Diabetic neuropathy represents a heterogeneous group of peripheral neuron disorders. It is distributed spatially (focal neuropathies, generalized neuropathies), temporally (reversible and persistent neuropathies), anatomically-clinically (neuropathy of sensitive, motor, and autonomic fibers, neuropathy of thin and thick fibers), microanatomically and histologically (axonal and demyelinating neuropathy).

Diabetic neuropathy is most often associated with motor-sensitive neuropathy almost in 70% of cases. It occurs most often on the lower limbs.

Diabetic neuropathy is a chronic, in most cases symmetrical, and fiber length-dependent polyneuropathy associated with long-term hyperglycemia. It affects all types of nerve fibers to varying degrees, initially manifesting as an impairment of sensitive fibers. Pain occurs in the later stages in the form of hypoesthesia or anesthesia. The process is chronic and progressive, lasting years. It is associated with diabetic retinopathy and nephropathy. Metabolic disorders triggered by hyperglycemia and microangiopathy are involved in the pathogenesis. The decisive factor in prevention and treatment is long-term and strict glycemic control.

From a practical clinical point of view, the classification into typical diabetic neuropathy and atypical diabetic neuropathy is currently preferred.

Table 11.1 Classification of Diabetic Neuropathy (Boulton, 2014)

1.	Subclinical (latent) neuropathy
2.	Clinical neuropathy
	Symmetric neuropathy
	Distal sensory-motor
	Acute painful neuropathy
	Diabetic autonomic neuropathy
	Hyperglycemic neuropathy
	Asymmetric (focal, multifocal) neuropathy
	Cranial
	Algic diabetic ophthalmoplegia
	Mononeuropathy IV, VI, and VII
	Peripheral mononeuropathies (median nerve, ulnar nerve, femoral nerve)
	Proximal diabetic amyotrophy (amyotrophic pelvic femoral syndrome)
	Thoracoabdominal algic neuropathy
	Mixed
	Combination of 2-3 types of neuropathies

Table 11.2 Another classification of Diabetic Neuropathy (Gilbey, 2004)

1.	**Rapidly reversible neuropathy**
	Hyperglycemic neuropathy
2.	**Persistent symmetrical neuropathy**
	Distal sensory-motor neuropathy with predominant impairment of thick fibers
	Autonomic neuropathy
	Thin fiber neuropathy
3.	**Focal/multifocal neuropathy**
	Cranial neuropathy
	Thoracoabdominal neuropathy
	Focal neuropathy of the limbs
	Proximal neuropathy
	Compressive and entrapment neuropathy

Typical diabetic neuropathy

It is a chronic, in most cases symmetrical, and fiber length-dependent polyneuropathy associated with long-term hyperglycemia. All nerve fibers are affected to varying degrees, with the initial manifestation of damage to sensitive fibers. Pain is more common in the later stages (hypesthesia to anesthesia). The course is chronic; it progresses over the years. Hyperglycemia-triggered metabolic disorder and microangiopathy are involved in the pathogenesis. The decisive factor in treatment is long-term strict glycemic control. It is often associated with retinopathy and nephropathy.

Atypical neurological neuropathy

They are rarer, affecting isolated cranial nerves, nerves of limbs and trunk, nerve plexuses, and roots. The onset is usually acute or subacute, and the course is monophasic, with fluctuating symptoms that subside within weeks or months. They preferentially affect thin fibers and are accompanied by pain and autonomic symptoms. The genesis is usually inflammatory and is not related to long-term hyperglycemia.

Distal symmetric sensory-motor neuropathy and its role in the pathogenesis of diabetic foot syndrome

It is the most common form and accounts for up to 2/3 of all diabetic feet. It is a diffusion process affecting sensitive motor and autonomic nerve fibers,

Table 11.3 Characteristics of typical and atypical diabetic neuropathy (Lobmann, 2011)

Typical diabetic neuropathy	Atypical diabetic neuropathy
Distal symmetric MS polyneuropathy	Focal and multifocal neuropathy
Chronic course	Acute, subacute, intercurrent, fluctuating, monophasic course
Lasting years	Duration of weeks, months
All fiber types are affected.	Thin fibers are preferentially affected.
Hypoesthesia/anesthesia, rare pain	Burning pain with hyperalgesia, autonomic symptoms
Long-term chronic hyperglycemia with a general metabolic disorder	Long-term hyperglycemia may not be present
Evidence of metabolic disorder and microangiopathy	Evidence for autoimmune inflammation
Association with diabetic nephropathy and retinopathy	Diabetic nephropathy and retinopathy are rare.
Prevention is the strict treatment of hyperglycemia.	

characterized by symmetrical impairment of the peripheral nerves of the limbs and trunk. The process is spread in the distal-proximal direction. However, if the limb is ischemic, it can also be an asymmetric disability. The long nerves of the lower limbs are usually affected first; symptoms appear on the thumbs and spread proximally, followed by symptoms on the upper limb, also directed proximally. Their onset is slow and gradual. They occur in both type 1 and type 2 diabetes, more often in older age and long duration of diabetes. In 50% of cases, it is asymptomatic. The first "positive" symptom is usually pain that appears in the evening, and at night, "negative" symptoms are also common: numbness, the feeling of a "wooden leg". It is accompanied by uncertainty when walking and standing (ataxia) due to impaired proprioceptive nerve fibers from joints, tendons, and muscles. If this symptom dominates, it is called ataxic neuropathy. Motor symptoms are less manifested. Instead, muscle fatigue appears after exertion and later atrophy of the leg's small muscles, which leads to a change in the configuration of the foot's arch. The sensation of alternating cold and heat is on the skin when the sympathetic fibers are affected. The skin is dry, non-sweating, and prone to rhagades. These symptoms arise independently of peripheral angiopathy. Patients observe hair loss characteristically in the innervation area of the fibular nerve on the foreleg, laterally from the edge of the tibia. If there is a loss of sensitive fibers for the perception of pain, touch, heat, and cold, the risk of imperceptible and painless leg trauma increases. Dysfunction of proprioceptive sensitive fibers from muscles, tendons, and joints changes the movement pattern of the foot stepping on the ground. When the arch of the foot changes, the point of contact of the foot with the ground changes, too. The function of the joints is uncoordinated; they are traumatized. The loss of motor fibers causes hypotrophy or atrophy of the small muscles of the leg and arch, which leads to a change in posture. Dysfunction of the autonomic sympathetic fibers innervating the sweat glands, regulating the trophicity of the skin and its adnexa, will cause a sweating disorder, thinning of the skin, and an increase in its vulnerability. Distal symmetrical sensory-motor neuropathy is, together with ischemia, a decisive risk factor for developing diabetic foot syndrome!

Painful forms of typical diabetic neuropathy

Acute painful diabetic neuropathy

It is a rare form. The clinical picture is dominated by pain and the presence of sensitive symptoms. It belongs to the group of neuropathies of thin nerve fibers. It occurs mainly in type 1 diabetes, with poor glycemic compensation or with rapid compensation of hyperglycemia - the so-called insulin neuritis. It is localized on the acral parts of the limbs, more prominently on the upper limbs. However, it may also appear more proximally and on the trunk. The pain is accentuated at night and during physical inactivity. It changes character (burning, cutting, prickly) and intensity (mild to unbearable) and is accompanied by dysesthesias (itching, burning, wood-leg syndrome, feeling of cold). It is characterized by hyperesthesia of the skin and allodynia caused by a gentle touch of the skin and hair (a light blanket). Loss of sensitivity is usually absent or minimal, as are motor symptoms. The onset is rapid; the prognosis is favorable, with adjustment over the course of months.

Chronic painful diabetic neuropathy

It is more frequent compared to the acute form. The incidence is reported to be 7-20%, twice as high in type 2 diabetes patients, with a 50% predominance of women. The occurrence of painful symptoms does not depend on the severity of neuropathy and insulin treatment. The clinical picture includes a spectrum of symptoms: tingling and burning to lancinating pain. Hyperalgesia and allodynia are present. The intensity of the symptoms is usually moderate to severe. The

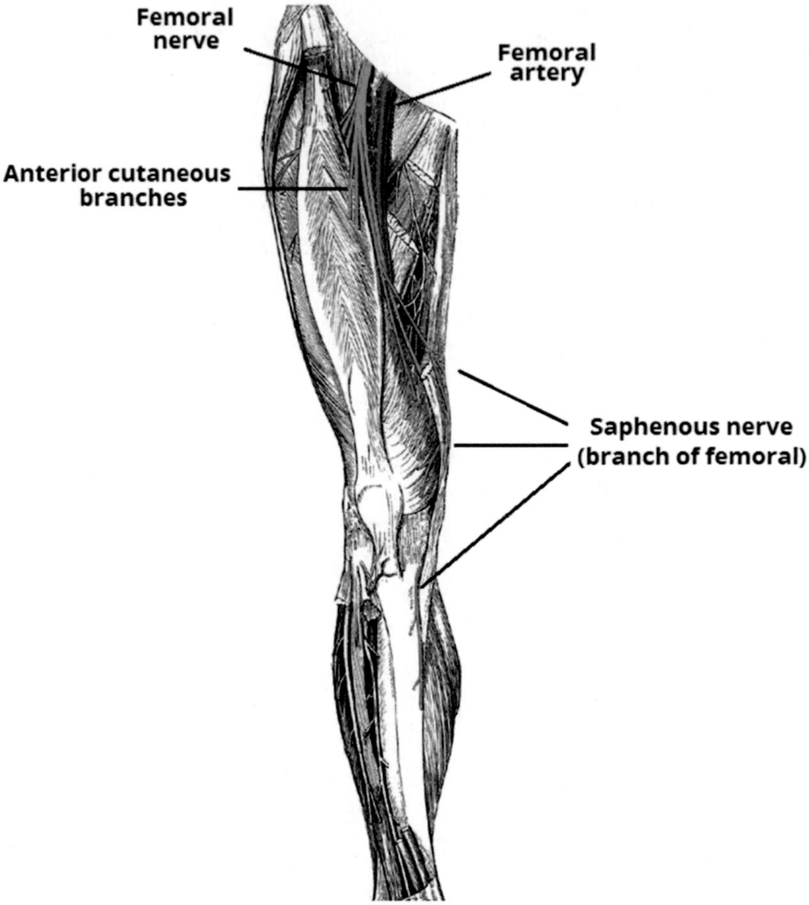

Figure 11.1 Innervation of the thigh (Gray anatomy).

distribution is also different: most often, the big toes and soles of the feet; if it spreads to the forelegs, the symptoms also begin to appear on the upper limbs. The prognosis of spontaneous adjustment is unfavorable, only in 23% of patients.

Clinical diagnosis and diagnostic criteria of neuropathy

Anamnesis

It is targeted at subjective symptoms from damage to sensitive, motor, and autonomic fibers, provoking moments, time patterns, manifestations,

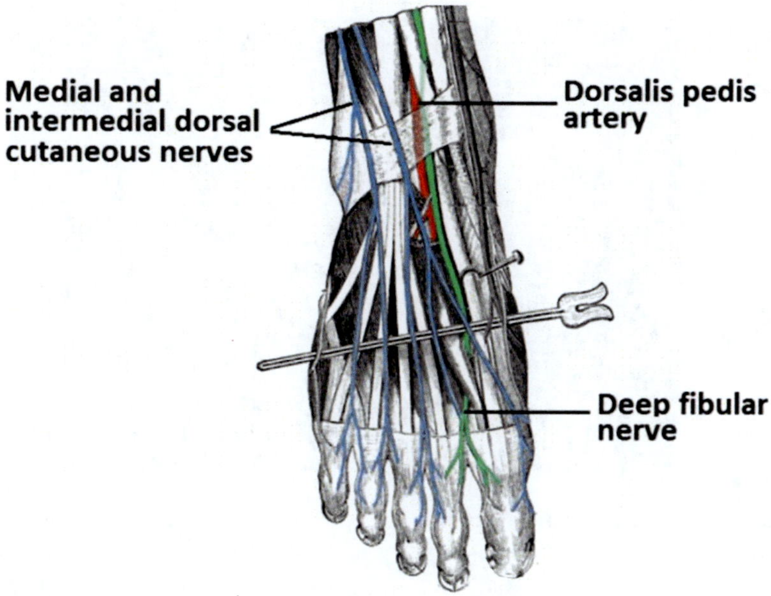

Figure 11.2 Innervation of the lower limb (source: Department of Vascular Surgery VUSCH).

quantification of pain, and intensity using simple scales. Purposely focus on hereditary neuropathies, exposure to toxic substances, presence of DM, prediabetes, and other metabolic, endocrine, and autoimmune diseases.

Observation and palpation

We record trophic changes in the skin, hair growth, temperature, humidity, skin color, muscle turgor, and muscle atrophy. We test the strength of muscle segments, posture stability, and walking with closed eyes.

Objective examination

We are focused on the function of thin and thick fibers. Sensory symptoms: paresthesia, dysesthesia, allodynia, pain. Motor symptoms: weakness, convulsions, fatigue. Autonomic symptoms: trophic changes in the skin, changes in blood circulation, and sweating of the skin.

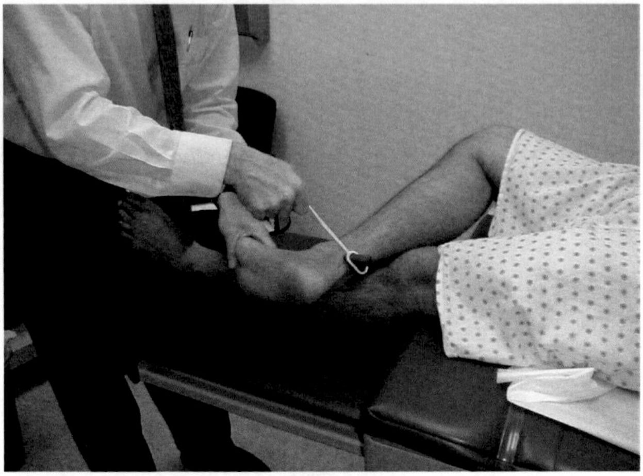

Figure 11.3 Clinical examination of the patient (source: Department of Vascular Surgery VUSCH).

Laboratory diagnostics

Table 11.4 Basic laboratory tests for neuropathies (Lobmann, 2011)

Hematological
Blood count
Sedimentation
CRP
Biochemical
Glycemia
oGTT
Markers of liver and renal functions
B12 vitamin
Malonic acid and homocysteine
Immunoelectrophoresis of serum proteins
Endocrine
Thyroid hormone level
Urine
Chemical examination
Glucose

Other examination methods

Direct methods show the nerve, and indirect ones reflect its function. MRI with the administration of a contrast agent is most often used for imaging,

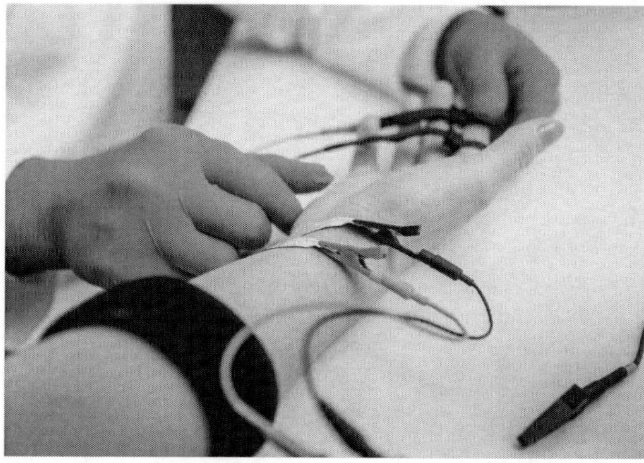

Figure 11.4 Electromyography (source: Department of Vascular Surgery VUSCH).

mainly to diagnose atypical neuropathies caused by nerve compression. Axon degeneration and secondary changes in the denervated muscle can be detected. Ultrasonography is also used (e.g., compression-carpal tunnel). Electromyography (EMG) is one of the indirect methods. It involves monitoring nerve and muscle function using an electromyographic device. This includes needle and stimulation EMG. Conductivity studies represent the gold standard in diagnostics; they are non-invasive, standardized, validated, and have high sensitivity and specificity. The results of their measurements are a sufficiently sensitive picture of the functional state of the sensory and motor fibers of the nerve. Examining nerves of the upper and lower limbs, which are accessible to contact surface stimulation, is standard.

References

Andersen H. Motor dysfunction in diabetes. Diabet. Metab. Res. Rev. 2012;28:89–92. doi: 10.1002/dmrr.2257.

Barker A.R., Rosson G.D., Dellon A.L. Wound healing in denervated tissue. Ann. Plast. Surg. 2006;57:339–342. doi: 10.1097/01.sap.0000221465.69826.b7.

Bentley J., Foster A. Multidisciplinary management of the diabetic foot ulcer. Br. J. Community Nurs. 2007;12:S6.

Boucek P. Advanced diabetic neuropathy—A point of no return? Rev. Diabet. Stud. 2006;3:143–150. doi: 10.1900/RDS.2006.3.143.

Boulton A.J. Diabetic neuropathy and foot complications. Handbook Clin. Neurol. 2014;126:97–107.

Boulton A.J. The diabetic foot: Grand overview, epidemiology, and pathogenesis. Diabet./Metab. Res. Rev. 2008;24:S3–S6. doi: 10.1002/dmrr.833.

Boulton A.J. The pathway to foot ulceration in diabetes. Med. Clin. N. Am. 2013;97:775–790. doi 10.1016/j.mcna.2013.03.007.

Boulton A.J. What you can't feel can hurt you. J. Vasc. Surg. 2010;52:28S–30S. doi: 10.1016/j.jvs.2010.06.005.

Boulton A.J., Kirsner R.S., Vileikyte L. Clinical practice. Neuropathic diabetic foot ulcers. N. Engl. J. Med. 2004;351:48–55. doi: 10.1056/NEJMcp032966.

Brandner J.M., Zacheja S., Houdek P., Moii I., Lobmann R. Expression of matrix metalloproteinases, cytokines, and connexins in diabetic and nondiabetic human keratinocytes before and after transplantation into an ex vivo wound-healing model. Diabet. Care. 2008;31:114–120. doi 10.2337/dc07-1304.

Broussard K.C., Powers J.G. Wound dressings: Selecting the most appropriate type. Am. J. Clin. Dermatol. 2013;14:449–459. Doi: 10.1007/s40257-013-0046-4.

Bruhn-Olszewska B., Korzon-Burakowska A., Gabig-Ciminska M., Olszewski P., Wegrzyn A., Jakobkiewicz-Banecka J. Molecular factors involved in the development of diabetic foot syndrome. Acta Biochim. Pol. 2012;59:507–513.

Cavanagh P.R., Bus S.A. Off-loading the diabetic foot for ulcer prevention and healing. Plast. Reconstr. Surg. 2011;127:248S–256S. doi: 10.1097/PRS.0b013e3182024864.

Cavanagh P.R., Bus S.A. Off-loading the diabetic foot for ulcer prevention and healing. J. Am. Podiatr. Med. Assoc. 2010;100:360–368. doi: 10.7547/1000360.

Da Silva L., Carvalho E., Cruz M.T. Role of neuropeptides in skin inflammation and its involvement in diabetic wound healing. Exp. Opin. Biol. Ther. 2010;10:1427–1439. doi 10.1517/14712598.2010.515207.

Dellon A.L. Susceptibility of nerve in diabetes to compression: Implications for pain treatment. Plast. Reconstr. Surg. 2014;134:142S–150S. doi: 10.1097/PRS.0000000000000668.

Dellon A.L., Muse V.L., Nickerson D.S. Prevention of ulceration, amputation, and reduction of hospitalization: Outcomes of a prospective multicenter trial of tibial neurolysis in patients with diabetic neuropathy. J. Reconstr. Microsurg. 2012;28:241–246. Doi: 10.1055/s-0032-1306372.

Generini S., Tuveri M.A., Matucci Cerinic M., Mastinu F., Manni L., Aloe L. Topical application of nerve growth factor in human diabetic foot ulcers. A study of three cases. Exp. Clin. Endocrinol. Diabet. Off. J. Ger. Soc. Endocrinol. Ger. Diabet. Assoc. 2004;112:542–544. doi: 10.1055/s-2004-821313.

Gilbey S.G. Neuropathy and foot problems in diabetes. Clin. Med. 2004;4:318–323. doi: 10.7861/clinmedicine.4-4-318.

Graiani G., Emanueli C., Desortes E., Linthout S.V., Pinna A., Figueroa C.D., Manni L., Nadeddu P. Nerve growth factor promotes reparative angiogenesis and inhibits endothelial apoptosis in cutaneous wounds of Type 1 diabetic mice. Diabetologia. 2004;47:1047–1054. doi 10.1007/s00125-004-1414-7.

Hochlenert D., Engels G. Integrated management in patients with diabetic foot syndrome. MMW Fortschr. Der Med. 2007;149:41–43.

Jeffcoate W.J. Wound healing—A practical algorithm. Diabet. Metab. Res. Rev. 2012;28:85–88. Doi: 10.1002/dmrr.2235.

Kamenov Z.A., Traykov L.D. Diabetic autonomic neuropathy. Adv. Exp. Med. Biol. 2012;771:176–193.

Kamenov Z.A., Traykov L.D. Diabetic somatic neuropathy. Adv. Exp. Med. Biol. 2012;771:155–175.

Krishnan S.T., Quattrini C., Jeziorska M., Malik R.A., Rayman G. Neurovascular factors in wound healing in the foot skin of type 2 diabetic subjects. Diabet. Care. 2007;30:3058–3062. doi 10.2337/dc07-1421.

Lobmann R. Diabetic foot syndrome. Der Internist. 2011;52:539–548. doi 10.1007/s00108-010-2733.

Lobmann R. Diabetic foot: How to avoid therapeutic mistakes. MMW Fortschr. Der Med. 2013;155:63–66. doi: 10.1007/s15006-013-2284.

Lobmann R., Achwerdov O., Brunk-Loch S., ENGELS G., Trocha A., Groene C., Kersken J. Diabetická noha v Nemecku 2005–2012: Analýza kvality v špecializovaných centrách starostlivosti o diabetickú nohu. Wound Med. 2014; 4 :27–29. Doi: 10.1016/j.wndm.2014.01.002.

Lobmann R., Ambrosch A., Schultz G., Waldmann K., Schiweck S., Lehnert H. Expression of matrix-metalloproteinases and their inhibitors in the wounds of diabetic and non-diabetic patients. Diabetologia. 2002;45:1011–1016. doi 10.1007/s00125-002-0868-8.

Lobmann R., Schultz G., Lehnert H. Proteases and the diabetic foot syndrome: Mechanisms and therapeutic implications. Diabet. Care. 2015;28:461–471. doi: 10.2337/diacare.28.2.461.

Molines L., Darmon P., Raccah D. Charcot's foot: Newest findings on its pathophysiology, diagnosis, and treatment. Diabet. Metab. 2010;36:251–255. doi 10.1016/j.diabet.2010.04.002.

Monteiro-Soares M., Boyko E.J., Ribeiro J., Dinis-Ribeiro L.M. Risk stratification systems for diabetic foot ulcers: A systematic review. Diabetologia. 2011;54:1190–1199. doi 10.1007/s00125-010-2030-3.

Morbach S., Muller E., Reike H., Risse A., Rumenapf G., Spraul M. Diabetic foot syndrome. Exp. Clin. Endocrinol. Diabet. Off. J. Ger. Soc. Endocrinol. Ger. Diabet. Assoc. 2014;122:416–424. doi: 10.1055/s-0034-1366455.

Motzkau M., Tautenhahn J., Lehnert H., Lobmann R. Expression of matrix-metalloproteases in the fluid of chronic diabetic foot wounds treated with a protease absorbent dressing. Exp. Clin. Endocrinol. Off. J. Ger. Soc. Endocrinol. Ger. Diabet. Assoc. 2011;119:286–290. doi: 10.1055/s-0030-1267235.

Mulder G., Tenenhaus M., D'souza G.F. Reduction of diabetic foot ulcer healing times through the use of advanced treatment modalities. Int. J. Low. Extreme. Wounds. 2014;13:335–346. doi 10.1177/1534734614557925.

Peltier A., Goutman S.A., Callaghan B.C. Painful diabetic neuropathy. BMJ. 2014;348:g1799. doi: 10.1136/bmj.g1799.

Pereira da Silva L., Miguel Neves B., Moura L., Cruz M.T., Eugenia C. Neurotensin decreases the proinflammatory status of human skin fibroblasts and increases epidermal growth factor expression. Int. J. Inflamm. 2014;2014:248240.

Rhim B., Harkless L. Prevention: Can we stop problems before they arise? Semin. Vasc. Surg. 2012;25:122–128. doi: 10.1053/j.semvascsurg.2012.05.002.

Risse A. Syndróm diabetickej nohy – interdisciplinárna výzva. Hamostaseológia. 2007; 27 :117-122.

Robinson C., Major M.J., Kuffel C., Hines K., Cole P. Orthotic management of the neuropathic foot: An interdisciplinary care perspective. Prosthet. Orthot. Int. 2015;39:73–81. doi 10.1177/0309364614545422.

Rumenapf G., Dittler S., Morbach S., Amendt K., Radu A. The vascular surgeon's role in interdisciplinary treatment of diabetic foot syndrome. Der Chir. Z. Fuer Alle Geb. Der Oper. Med. 2008;79:535–545.

Russell J.W., Zilliox L.A. Diabetic neuropathies. Continuum. 2014;20:1226–1240. doi 10.1212/01.CON.0000455884.29545.d2.

Said G. Diabetic neuropathy. Handbook Clin. Neurol. 2013;115:579–589.

Sandireddy R., Yerra V.G., Areti A., Komirishetty P., Kumar A. Neuroinflammation and oxidative stress in diabetic neuropathy: Futuristic strategies based on these targets. Int. J. Endocrinol. 2014;2014:674987. doi 10.1155/2014/674987.

Shalaby S.Y., Blume P., Sumpio B.E. New modalities in the chronic ischemic diabetic foot management. Clin. Podiatr. Med. Surg. 2014;31:27–42. doi: 10.1016/j.cpm.2013.09.009.

Singh V.P., Bali A., Singh N., Jaggi A.S. Advanced glycation end products and diabetic complications. Korean J. Physiol. Pharmacol. 2014;18:1–14. doi: 10.4196/kjpp.2014.18.1.1.

Soliman M., Rajbhandari S.M. Assessing outcome of diabetic foot ulcers and multidisciplinary foot clinic. Curr. Diabet. Rev. 2013;9:397–401. doi: 10.2174/15733998113099990075.

Tavee J., Zhou L. Small fiber neuropathy: A burning problem. Clevel. Clin. J. Med. 2009;76:297–305. doi: 10.3949/ccjm.76a.08070.

Tiaka E.K., Papanas N., Manolakis A.C., Maltezos E. The role of nerve growth factor in the prophylaxis and treatment of diabetic foot ulcers. Int. J. Burn. Trauma. 2011;1:68–76.

Van Battum P., Schaper N., Prompers L., Apelqvist J., Jude E. Differences in minor amputation rate in diabetic foot disease throughout Europe are in part explained by differences in disease severity at presentation. Diabet. Med. J. Br. Diabet. Assoc. 2011;28:199–205. doi: 10.1111/j.1464-5491.2010.03192.

Vinik A.I., Maser R.E., Mitchell B.D., Freeman R. Diabetic autonomic neuropathy. Diabet. Care. 2003;26:1553–1579. doi: 10.2337/diacare.26.5.1553.

Wukich D.K., Armstrong D.G., Attinger C.E., Boulton A.J.M., Burns P.R., Frykberg R.G., Hellman R., Kim P.J., Lipsky B.A., Piel J.C., et al. Inpatient management of diabetic foot disorders: A clinical guide. Diabet. Care. 2013;36:2862–2871. doi 10.2337/dc12-2712.

Zenker J., Ziegler D., Chrast R. Novel pathogenic pathways in diabetic neuropathy. Trends Neurosci. 2013;36:439–449. doi: 10.1016/j.tins.2013.04.008.

Ziegler D., Keller J., Maier C., Pannek J. Diabetic neuropathy. Exp. Clin. Endocrinol. Diabet. Off. J. Ger. Soc. Endocrinol. Ger. Diabet. Assoc. 2014;122:406–415. doi: 10.1055/s-0034-1366435.

A., Reeps C., Hartl F., Ockert S., Eckstein H.H. The diabetic foot. Der Chir. Z. Fuer Alle Geb. Der Oper. Med. 2009;80:430–436.

Chapter 12

Chronic Pain in Peripheral Artery Disease

Martina Zavacká, MD*

Department of Vascular Surgery, East Slovak Institute of Cardiovascular Diseases, Faculty of Medicine, Pavol Jozef Šafárik University in Košice, Slovakia

Abstract

Pain is an unpleasant emotional and sensory experience associated with potential or actual tissue damage. Chronic pain is so complex that it can only be solved with a multidisciplinary approach. In recent years, its importance has grown so much that it forced the creation of a new medical discipline - algesiology. Individual patients perceive pain differently and attribute a different meaning to it. Therefore, post-operative and post-traumatic pain treatment improves patient comfort, reduces physical and psychological stress, and improves patient motivation and mobility. Thus, recovery is accelerated.

Key Words: pain, algesiologist, comfort, stress, opioids

Definition and Etiology of Pain

"Pain is an unpleasant sensation or emotional experience associated with actual or potential tissue damage or described in terms of such damage," says the definition of pain proposed by the International Association for the Study of Pain. IASP defines pain as an unpleasant emotional and sensory experience associated with potential or actual tissue damage.

Loeser's model explains the essence of pain, which understands it as a complex of physiological and psychological factors. Pain is also the most

* Corresponding Author's Email: martina.zavacka@upjs.sk

In: Diabetic Foot
Editor: Martina Zavacká
ISBN: 979-8-89113-019-7

common symptom of why a patient consults a doctor. In recent years, its importance has grown so much that it forced the creation of a new medical discipline - algesiology and doctors - algesiologists. Pain is always subjective, yet it remains a subject of interest to physicians of all fields. The algesiologist acquires a dominant role, mainly in treating cancer and chronic pain. Chronic pain is so complex that it can only be effectively addressed with a multidisciplinary approach. Each team member contributes with their knowledge and skills to achieve the common goal - the correct diagnosis of pain and the determination of the most effective therapeutic procedure.

The different perception of pain is explained by the individual and distinct perception of pain and the meaning that individuals attribute to it. This meaning includes a complex of psychological, emotional, cultural-social interactions and biological factors. Previous positive or negative experiences of pain treatment also influence manifestations of pain. The level of perceived pain is affected by these factors: fear, anxiety, the ability of the patient to control the pain and the ability to rise above the pain, the perception of the strategy and attitudes of the nursing staff, and the reactions and responses of other patients to pain. Acute pain occurs in the post-traumatic and postoperative periods or during acute exacerbation of chronic diseases.

Clinical division of pain and the need for its control

The pain has a rapid onset - a phasic component and a tonic component of varying duration. This is one of the factors by which we distinguish between acute and chronic pain. However, they are two different units, and their meaning for the patient and the doctor is also different (Table 12.1). Today, it is generally accepted that uncontrolled pain adversely affects patients and their families.

Table 12.1 Intensity and duration of postoperative pain (Rokyta, 1995)

Location of surgery	Need for opiates (h)	Pain VAS
Thoracotomy	72-96	10
Upper abdomen	48-72	7-8
Lower abdomen	<48	5
Hip joint	<48	5
Faciomaxillary	<48	5
Perineum	24-48	5
Limbs	24-36	5
Skin	<24	5
Inguinal - herniotomy	<36	2-3

Treatment of acute pain

According to the location of reactivity to a painful stimulus, we can divide the individual levels of pain manifestations into the following:

1. Segmental level (muscle tension, O2, lactate)
2. Suprasegmental level (sympathicotonia)
3. Cortical level (fear and anxiety)

Negative effects of pain

A) Neurohumoral effects of pain. The production of catabolic hormones (ACTH, cortisol, catecholamines, ADH, aldosterone, renin, cAMP) increases. The production of anabolic hormones (insulin, testosterone) decreases.
B) Respiratory consequences of pain. The functional residual capacity of the lungs (FRC), the vital capacity of the lungs (VC), the compliance of the chest, the rate of forced exhalation (FEV1), and expectoration decrease. Hypoxemia, atelectasis, and even bronchopneumonia develop.
C) Circulatory effects of pain. Sympathicotonia accelerates and burdens the activity of the cardiovascular system. There is an increased risk of various disorders in ischemic heart disease. If the patient's mobility during rehabilitation is not sufficient, there is a risk of thrombosis and the development of thromboembolic disease.
D) Effect of pain on the gastrointestinal tract. Pain is involved in developing postoperative nausea and vomiting (PONV). Even paralytic ileus is more pronounced with pain than without it.
E) Urogenital system. Pain negatively affects bladder motility and micturition kinetics.

Pain has many adverse effects on the body, often with fatal consequences. The diagnostic and informative significance of pain can be overcome in the current era of the existence of other modern diagnostic techniques. Therefore, it is possible and indicated to treat the pain. According to some reasoned rules, "freedom from pain should be one of the basic human rights." Therefore, the anesthesiologist and every healthcare worker should be familiar with the basic pain treatment methods.

Postoperative and post-traumatic pain treatment improves patient comfort, reduces physical and psychological stress, and improves the motivation and mobility of the patient. Therefore, recovery is accelerated. Adequate treatment can also prevent the development of chronic neuropathic pain if the disease becomes chronic.

The anesthesiologist is in an ideal position for postoperative analgesia because he has tested the patient's reactivity to pain during anesthesia.

Intensity and duration of postoperative pain

The intensity and duration of postoperative pain are influenced by the location, extent, and duration of the operation, the size of the surgical wound (including the extent of the skin incision), the patient's attitude towards the operation, the method of preoperative preparation (premedication, preemptive analgesia, etc.), the possible occurrence of postoperative surgical complications and perioperative anesthesia care. Despite certain principles, the feeling and interpretation of pain are strictly individual. Therefore, estimating pain intensity should be developed individually, considering the interaction of various factors.

A simple aid is also used for this - the pain visual analog scale (VAS), which will help us to make the pain "visible" to a certain extent. Maintaining acute pain intensity with treatment at a value of 3 or less is currently recommended. Chronic pain intensity should not reach 3, with a maximum value of 2.

Methods of treatment of postoperative pain

1. Traditional local intramuscular administration of opiates
2. Intravenous administration of opiates (boluses, continuous, PCA)
3. Other administration of opiates (oral, rectal, subcutaneous, transdermal, nasal, neuraxial, intra-articular)
4. Use of local anesthetics (local, spinal, epidural)
5. Nonsteroidal anti-inflammatory drugs (NSAIDs)
6. Alpha2 mimetics (systemic, epidural)
7. Non-pharmacological methods (cryotherapy, transcutaneous electrostimulation – TENS, acupuncture, psychological methods)

Analgesia dosing intervals

Dosing intervals of analgesic drugs also significantly affect the success of pain treatment. With long intervals between doses, patients actively report significant pain, and their traumatization is more significant. With optimal intervals, the patient is without significant pain for a long time.

Morphine is a classic opiate. Despite the availability of many other opiates with unique properties superior to morphine, it still has its place in algesiology. Its continuous intravenous application is also used, but this method is reserved only for intensive care units, especially for patients with artificial ventilation.

Patient Controlled Analgesia (PCA)

It is performed with a syringe pump, in which a syringe with an analgesic mixture is inserted. The pump is connected to the patient via an infusion line (intravenous or epidural). The patient has a push-button switch in his hand, connected to the pump by a cable. At the onset of pain, the patient can self-administer a dose of painkiller by pressing the switch. The pump is adjusted so the patient cannot overdose by repeatedly pressing the button. This is done by setting a non-corresponding time interval on the pump. The pump can also set the administration of a basal analgesic dose, which is independent of the dosing activity of the patient.

The advantages of such treatment are the possibility of regulating the treatment by the patient (the pharmacodynamic differences of the specific patient are respected), low doses are applied with minor changes in the blood levels of the analgesic with a reduction in the occurrence of its undesirable effects, it relieves the nurse of a burden, the application is painless, and the placebo

Table 12.2 Properties of morphine (Ševčík, 1994)

Analgesia	Constipation, nausea, and vomiting
Breathing depression	Miosis
Sedation	Spasms of the bile ducts
Antitussive	Urinary retention
Vasodilatation	Tolerance
Release of histamine	Habit

Table 12.3 Intravenous administration of opiates (Rokyta, 1995)

Advantages	Disadvantages
Rapid onset of analgesia	Fixed dose without relation to pharmacodynamic variability
Balanced plasma levels	The fatality of errors
Painless delivery	Expensive monitoring
NCA (nurse-controlled analgesia) pump	Reduction of nurses' attention

effect of the patient's will is not negligible (some of the patient's button compressions are without the application response of the pump and the patient does not know which compression was followed by the application of the analgesic).

The disadvantage is the fatality of possible technical errors of the device, its high price, and the need for cooperation and understanding of the patient, which is sometimes impossible to achieve in practice.

Other routes of administration of opiates

Sublingual: It requires patient cooperation; only buprenorphine is administered this way.

Oral: It is unsuitable for postoperative analgesia, it has delayed absorption, and there is a possibility of the accumulation of analgesics in the digestive system; the first-pass effect applies to morphine, so dihydrocodeine and NSAIDs can be administered in the later postoperative period.

Rectal: The disadvantage is the plasma level variability; it bypasses the portal vein, and the advantage is avoiding absorption disorders from the upper part of the gastrointestinal tract.

Transdermal: The substance must be fat-soluble; this route of application is more suitable for the treatment of chronic pain, not acute, e.g., fentanyl.

Local anesthetics (in a single dose or through a catheter)

A local anesthetic is a medicine that blocks the conduction of nerve impulses from the site of injury so that pain signals are not transmitted to the brain. Normal nerve impulses require the opening of sodium channels in the nerve cell membrane. The influx of sodium ions into the nerve fiber causes its depolarization, which spreads along the nerve fiber. The local anesthetic temporarily closes the sodium channels in the nerve cell membrane.

Places of administration of local anesthetics in the treatment of pain:

- Subarachnoid anesthesia
- Epidural anesthesia, caudal block
- Intercostal block, intrapleural analgesia
- Peripheral block, plexus blocks
- Incisional analgesia

The advantage of administering local anesthetics is avoiding the undesirable effects of opiates, such as nausea and respiratory depression. The disadvantage is the blockade of nerve transmission at higher doses (weakness of the lower limbs, micturition disorder) and vasodilation from sympathetic blockade (drop in blood pressure). This technique can provide analgesia continually via a catheter after a procedure/surgery performed with local anesthesia.

Analgesia with local anesthetics is excellent, especially in the early postoperative phase. For example, a "single shot" dose of bupivacaine administered epidurally has an analgetic effect for 4 to 6 hours and a peripheral block for up to 8 to 18 hours! When adjuvant substances such as adrenaline or clonidine are added, the duration of analgesia is even longer. We can use the catheter technique to maintain analgesia with local anesthetics for many days.

Postoperative epidural analgesia continues after epidural anesthesia or combined anesthesia (general + epidural anesthesia by catheter technique). The catheter is introduced near the segment with maximal pain. The injection site during surgery in the lower abdomen is at the level of T9, and in the upper abdomen T6, there is seven times less morphine consumption. Still, even here, respiratory depression is possible. Undesirable motor block of the lower limbs, when the catheter is inserted above L2, occurs in 1%, after lower insertion of the catheter below L2 in up to 33%.

Complications of neuraxial analgesia

- Hypotension (hypovolemia, sympatholysis, reducing the amount of local anesthetic)
- Motor block (do not administer in the unconscious state; administer more cranially if a block of the lower limbs is not desired)
- Intense sensitive block (watch out for pressure ulcers)
- Urinal retention (even with local anesthetics and opiates)
- Epidural hematoma (1:11000, dg. up to 8h, paresis/plegia with preserved sensitivity)
- Epidural abscess paresis (paresis/plegia with preserved sensitivity, fevers)

NSAIDs

NSAIDs (non-steroidal anti-inflammatory drugs) can be used as a complementary therapy in minor surgical procedures. They reduce the use of opioids. They relieve pain even 24-48 hours after surgery. However, their use is associated with specific problems, such as causing ulcers and worsening the function of the kidneys and blood platelets, especially in unstable and high-risk postoperative patients. In addition, they are considered unsuitable for the treatment of severe pain.

Potential complications of NSAID use:

- Renal failure
- Bronchospasms

- Increased bleeding
- Ulcerogenic effect
- Local pain at the injection site/tissue necrosis

Examples of NSAIDs used for postoperative analgesia:

- for oral administration: paracetamol and codeine,
- for rectal administration: paracetamol, diclofenac, and metamizole,
- for intramuscular administration: diclofenac, metamizole and ketoprofen,
- for intravenous administration: ketoprofen and diclofenac.

Postoperative pain treatment combined with analgesia (protocol)

- Paracetamol supp. 1 g/6 hours rectally
- Mixture of bupivacaine 0.25% with adrenaline 1:200,000 50 ml + sufentanil 50 mg by pump 2-8 ml/h epidurally
- In case of pain, administer a bolus of the mixture mentioned above
- In case of acute pain, administer opiate intravenously
- Monitoring: pain VAS (1-10), BP, P, D (count and paCO2), dermatome, sedation monitoring (Ramsay score 1-6), motor block monitoring (Bromage scale 1-3), patient satisfaction assessment (marks like at school)
- Permanent availability: anesthesiologist, intravenous access, crystalloid, ephedrine, atropine, naloxone, oxygen, metoclopramide...

Preemptive analgesia

The administration of analgesics before nociceptive stimulation attempts to prevent CNS sensitization and hyperpathic processing of the nociceptive stimulus (hyperalgesia). NSAID, opiates, regional anesthesia, and ketamine are used.

Teams for the treatment of acute pain (Acute Pain Service, APS)

In hospitals, they ensure the effectiveness, availability, and monitoring of pain treatment. The Acute Pain Service (APS) includes a multidisciplinary approach to pain management. It consists of anesthesiologists, nurses, and other medical and healthcare staff to optimize the treatment of postoperative pain. APS necessarily requires anesthesiologists.

Composition of the APS team:

- anesthesiologist (pain specialist)
- nurse anesthetist

(implementation, documentation, evaluation, application, communication...)

- anesthesiologist specialized in the relevant workplace
- primary care physician
- nurses of the primary care
- nurses of primary care on duty
- nurse anesthetist on duty

The nurse closest to the patient has a key and unique role in assessing and treating postoperative pain.

Chronic pain

It may begin acutely but persists long after the damage has ended. Neural mechanisms intervene here, which are much more complex than during acute pain. The motivational-affective dimension of pain comes to the fore more. The course is cyclical and often worsens, and we cannot predict the end; if adaptation of the autonomic nervous system has occurred and objective symptoms are absent. When it remains uncontrolled, it becomes the meaning of the patient's life, disturbs his sleep and appetite, and worsens relationships at the workplace and in the family; organic depression affects up to 25% of patients. Regardless of whether the cause is known or the pain is present without an apparent organic reason, chronic pain ceases to be a symptom of a disease and becomes an independent disease.

Pathophysiological division of pain

The stimulation of nociceptors causes nociceptive pain. According to the location of nociceptors, superficial (skin and mucous membranes), deep (somatic) - coming from the musculoskeletal system, and visceral pain is distinguished.

Neuropathic (neurogenic) pain originates from peripheral or central nervous system lesions. The pain can be paroxysmal, sharp, pricking, strong, shooting-neuralgic or permanent, mild to moderate intensity, burning, unpleasant - deafferentation. Qualitative and quantitative sensory changes are present at the same time.

Pain scales
Numerical pain scale 0 1 2 3 4 5 6 7 8 9 10
Pain Visual Analogue Scale (VAS)

Classification of pain based on neuropathophysiological mechanisms is crucial for treatment tactics. While primary analgesics are effective for nociceptive pain, neuropathic pain is more or less resistant, and secondary analgesics play a dominant role here.

Table 12.4 PQRST pain characteristic (Striebel, 1993)

P Pain localization; Where does it hurt?
Q Quality of the pain; What is the pain like?
R Radiation of the pain; Is it spreading somewhere?
S Severity (intensity) of the pain; How strong is the pain?
T Time duration; Is the pain constant, or does it change?
Precipitating(provoking) factors; What makes the pain worse?
Relief factors; What relieves the pain?

Diagnosis of the cause of pain

It is essential for a rational treatment procedure. The prerequisite is obtaining an adequate anamnesis of the felt pain in pathophysiological terms (nociceptive, neuropathic), taking into account the intensity of the pain and assessing the presence of psycho-social factors, a general physical examination and an examination of the location of the pain. It should be remembered that pain is always subjective; no neuropsychological or chemical test can be used to measure it. A helpful aid in determining the cause of pain is the description of pain using the PQRST characteristic (Table 12.4). Visual analog, verbal and numerical scales are used to determine pain intensity, and their use is further extended to assess pain relief concerning prescribed treatment.

Pharmacotherapy of pain

The basis is a systematic pharmacological procedure based on three groups of drugs: Non-opioid analgesics, opioid analgesics, and adjuvant drugs - secondary analgesics. They are used according to pain intensity and are known as a three-step analgesic ladder, recommended by the World Health Organization.

It takes into account five basic principles of analgesic application in chronic cancer pain:

a) orally
b) according to hours (regular dosing interval, not in case of pain)
c) according to the ascending ladder
d) the dose is individually titrated against the patient's pain
e) we pay attention to details

Table 12.5 Three-step analgesic ladder (Klener, 1995)

I. non-opioid analgesics +/-adjuvant drugs
II. opioids for mild and moderate pain +/- non-opioid analgesics +/- adjuvant medications
III. opioids for moderate and severe pain +/- non-opioid analgesics +/- adjuvant medications

Non-opioid analgesics (step I)

They are intended for mild to moderate intensity pain of any etiology. They are particularly suitable for the pain of musculoskeletal origin; they are the drug of first choice for bone metastases. It is a chemically diverse group of primary analgesics:

1. Nonsteroidal anti-inflammatory drugs (NSAIDs) work by inhibiting the cyclooxygenase enzyme, which catalyzes arachidonic acid's conversion to prostaglandins and leukotrienes. They are primarily used to control inflammatory pain and as co-analgesics. The limiting factor is the number of adverse effects: nephrotoxicity, hepatotoxicity, hemocoagulation disorders, gastropathy to gastroduodenal ulceration, headaches, tinnitus, states of confusion, edema, and urticaria. Adverse effects are more frequent and more severe with chronic application. Short-term effective forms and preparations with a more favorable COX1/COX2 ratio are preferable for treating chronic pain with long-acting drugs of this group. Ibuprofen is the drug of the first choice among NSAIDs. Alternatives are diclofenac (in combination with misoprostol), flurbiprofen, naproxen, ketoprofen, meloxicam, nimesulide, nabumetone, and indomethacin.
2. Acetylsalicylic acid, unlike other substances of this group, causes irreversible inhibition of the cyclooxygenase pathway and has more pronounced side effects on the GIT and hemocoagulation. Non-acetylated salicylates such as lysine salicylate have smaller effects on hemocoagulation.
3. Paracetamol (acetaminophen) is the analgesic of the first choice from this group. The advantage is that it does not affect the function of platelets, so it is safe even in patients with thrombocytopenia. At the used dosage of 500-1000 mg every 4-6 hours, it has no adverse effects on the GIT; higher dosages are limited by hepatotoxicity.
4. Metamizole has an excellent analgesic and antipyretic effect and is antiphlogistic in higher doses. The main advantage is its spasmolytic effect, which is also used to control visceral and neuropathic pain. The limitation is the impact on hematopoiesis, allergic reactions, porphyria, and liver and kidney insufficiency.

Recommended procedure:

a) The choice of the most appropriate analgesic from this group depends on the patient's tolerance; in case of intolerance to one preparation, it can be replaced by another, and the combination of several drugs from the same group is not recommended.
b) Non-opioid analgesics have a synergistic effect with the central effect of opioids, i.e., opioid-sparing effect. Combination with opioids is advantageous.
c) Their use is limited by the ceiling effect (i.e., low analgesic potential); increasing the dose above a certain level does not increase the analgesic effect, only the adverse side effects.
d) The maximum doses are 1.5–2 times the standard doses.
e) In case of persistent pain, we do not prolong the application of non-opioid analgesics alone but choose a combination with analgesics of higher levels of the analgesic ladder.

Opioid analgesics

Opioids are the largest group of primary analgesics used to control mild, moderate, and severe pain due to their effectiveness, easy titration, and excellent risk/benefit ratio. Analgesia is a consequence of binding with specific opioid receptors in the CNS and the periphery. Activation of receptors in the periaqueductal gray matter and spinal cord causes analgesia, and activation of receptors in other levels of the CNS and in the periphery causes euphoria, respiratory depression, sedation, constipation, nausea, and urinary retention. Opioids are divided into the following groups:

A) pure agonists (codeine, dihydrocodeine, oxycodone, tilidine, tramadol, pethidine, piritramide, morphine, fentanyl, methadone) do not have a ceiling effect of analgesic efficacy, do not antagonize the effects of other opioids when administered simultaneously.
B) partial agonists (buprenorphine) have relatively low intrinsic activity when binding with opioid receptors and, compared to pure agonists, have a ceiling effect of analgesia.
C) mixed agonists/antagonists (pentazocine, butorphanol, nalbuphine) have a ceiling effect of analgesic efficacy; in contrast to pure agonists, they cause analgesia on one receptor (m) and at the same time neutralize it on another receptor (k). Simultaneous application of pure agonists and mixed agonists/antagonists induces a withdrawal syndrome and increases pain.

Opioid analgesics for mild and moderate pain – step II.
Among the analgesics that are included in this group (Table 12.6), the following are currently used to control cancer pain:

1. Codeine and dihydrocodeine (the latter is available in a timed-release form) are partially bio-transformed into morphine and act as "weak morphine"; a significant antitussive effect is also advantageous. When increasing the dose above the average therapeutic level (more than 200 mg per day), there is a proportionally higher incidence of adverse effects (constipation), which limit their use.
2. Tramadol is a synthetic opioid that acts as a pure agonist; inhibiting noradrenaline and serotonin reuptake also participates in the mechanism of its analgesic effect, which extends its indication to neuropathic pain. It does not cause spasms of the sphincter of Oddi and does not change bile secretion. It has a range of forms: tablets, capsules, drops, suppositories, and injections; it is also available in a timed-release form.
3. Alternatives are tilidine and buprenorphine.
4. Other opioids of this group, such as piritramide, butorphanol, and nalbuphine, are only in parenteral form and are therefore not recommended for chronic pain control.

Table 12.6 Overview of some recommended non-opioid analgesics (Jacox et al., 1994)

generic name	a single dose (mg)	dosing interval (hours)	max. recommended dose (mg/day)
paracetamol	500 - 1000	4-6	4000
acetylsalicylic acid	500 - 1000	4-6	4000
ibuprofen	400	6	2400
diclofenac	25-100	8	200
diclofenac/misoprostol	50/0.2	12	200/0.8
ketoprofen	25	8	200
flubiprofen	100	12	300
indomethacin	25 - 100	12	200
naproxen	250	12	1000
diflunisal	500	12	1500
meloxicam	7.5	24	15
nimesulide	100	12	400
nabumetone	500	24	2000
piroxicam	20	24	40
metamizole	500 - 1000	4-6	6000

5. Absolutely unsuitable for the treatment of chronic cancer pain, evaluated as a "non-lege artis" procedure are:
   Pethidine (meperidine) due to short effect (2-3h) and poor bioavailability after oral application. With the chronic application, in higher doses and elderly patients, its metabolite normeperidine accumulates, which has a toxic effect on the CNS, causing tremors, convulsions, and agitation.
   Pentazocine due to the short duration of action, the unreliability of oral administration, the rapid onset of addiction, and significant psychomimetic effects.

Opioid analgesics for moderate and severe pain – step III.

Morphine is the opioid of choice for moderate to severe pain. The initial dose is calculated using an equivalent conversion. The dose is titrated until pain relief is achieved, and there is no maximum dose. 90% of patients with morphine-sensitive pain often do not need a higher daily dose than 200-300 mg, but individual doses may be 1000 times higher. Usability in the body varies from 35-75% during oral administration; with chronic administration, the oral/parenteral ratio is 2:1 to 3:1. The combination of morphine with weak and strong opioid agonists is illogical. The classic Brompton mixture and ethylmorphine pills are now considered obsolete. Combination with partial opioid agonists and mixed agonists/antagonists is unacceptable.

Adverse effects of opioids

When treating with opioids, it is necessary to pay attention to their adverse effects; the occurrence is very variable, and careful monitoring and prophylactic treatment are required.

The most common side effect of the long-term opioid application is constipation; tolerance is very slow or absent. Increasing the intake of liquids and

Table 12.7 Opioids for mild and moderate pain – step II (Kočan et al., 2015)

generic name	oral dose (mg)	dosing interval (hours)
dihydrocodeine	60-120	12
oxycodone	5 - 10	4 - 6
tilidine	50 - 100	4
tramadol	50 - 100	4-6
buprenorphine	0.4	8
pethidine	50 - 100	2 - 3
pentazocine	50 - 100	2 - 3

fibers is enough as a preventive measure in case of mild symptoms. In case of severe symptoms, it is necessary to include laxatives: irritant stimulants - bisacodyl, senna, osmotic - lactulose, and prokinetics of the digestive tract (cisapride).

Sedation – is temporary when increasing the dose of opioids; tolerance occurs in 5-7 days. Persistent sedation requires reducing the dose or extending the interval of opioid administration and administering CNS stimulants: caffeine, phenmetrazine, pyritinol, and piracetam.

Nausea and vomitus – the treatment depends on the underlying cause; neuroleptics prochlorperazine, perphenazine, haloperidol, and droperidol are effective, and if they fail, antiemetics, metoclopramide, ondansetron should be used.

Depression of breathing - pain is a physiological antagonist of the respiratory depressant effect of opioids. Respiratory depression does not occur when the patient is receiving the correct doses of opioids for pain control. As long as pain exists, the dose of morphine can be safely titrated upwards without concern about respiratory depression.

Tolerance to opioids is defined as the need to increase the dose to achieve the previous analgesic effect. We can prevent tolerance to a certain extent:

- by using a combination of opioids and non-opioids
- by an appropriate alternation of strong opioids, as the cross-tolerance between them is not complete
- by favoring oral administration over parenteral routes, since tolerance, as a function of dose and frequency of administration, occurs more quickly with intravenous infusions.

Physical dependence manifests itself as a withdrawal syndrome when opioids are stopped suddenly. Withdrawal syndrome is a function of opioid half-life, for morphine and short-half-life opioids developing after 6-12 hours, with a peak after 24-72 hours. It does not happen if we reduce the doses gradually over 3-5 days. For opioids with a long half-life (transdermal fentanyl), the syndrome is delayed by 24 hours. Withdrawal syndrome can sometimes be considered a viral disease, flu, or "flu-like" syndrome (cough, lacrimation, colic, diarrhea).

Addiction (i.e., psychological dependence) refers to a specific drug-induced mood that associates drug use with a good and desirable feeling. The use of opioids for a medical indication is very rarely related to the development of addiction.

Other side effects, such as urinary retention or pruritus, can be addressed by changing the opioid, changing the route of administration, or using an opioid antagonist – naloxone, in slowly titrated doses that do not antagonize analgesia.

Adjuvant drugs

They are a large group of drugs that increase the effectiveness of primary analgesics, treat accompanying symptoms that increase pain, show their independent analgesic activity in specific types of pain, and also reduce the undesirable effects of anesthetics. They are used at every step of the analgesic ladder.

Corticosteroids effectively treat inflammatory pain (e.g., bone pain), neuropathic pain, and headaches due to intracranial hypertension. They reduce brain and spinal cord edema and relieve pain caused by perineural edema and oppression of peripheral nerves. They reduce nausea, increase appetite and improve mood. They are especially beneficial for cachectic patients with terminal cancer, increasing their quality of life and a general sense of health. Anticonvulsants are used to control sharp, shooting neuralgic pain.

Antidepressants are the first-choice pain treatment for continuous dysesthesia (burning) pain; their antidepressant effect and sleep improvement are also used for cancer pain.

Neuroleptics have an additive analgesic effect, and their antiemetic and antipsychotic impact is significant. They potentiate the effect of antidepressants; the extraordinary thing is that the pain loses its affective charge.

Anxiolytics are used on a limited and short-term basis for cancer pain: acute procedural pain and terminal anxiety.

Hypnotics are not recommended alone because they fail in severe pain. A combination of analgesics and psychopharmaceuticals is suitable.

Psychostimulants have an additive analgesic effect and a centrally stimulating effect on the sedative effect of opioids. They are rarely used, and their indication increases with narcolepsy.

Calcitonin and bisphosphonates (pamidronate, clodronate) are analgesics in primary or secondary hormone-independent bone metastases and osteoporotic pain due to metabolic or other reasons.

Spasmoanalgesics relieve biliary and renal colic pain and are used in colicky visceral pain and GIT obstruction.

Central myorelaxants are used for musculoskeletal pain.

Physical therapy

- Exercise and rehabilitation procedures (massages, application of heat, cold, electro-, and hydrotherapy) targeted concerning the patient's condition and protection against possible damage.

- Lifestyle changes, immobilization, and various orthopedic aids are helpful for patients whose pain increases with movement.
- TENS - transcutaneous electrical neurostimulation and acupuncture can benefit some patients initially.

Psychosocial interventions

- Psychotherapeutic and relaxation techniques
- Patient education must be a part of pain treatment. Because many myths about pain and its treatment persist, it is necessary to explain the essence of pain understandably, inform about the possibilities of its effective control, and disprove unjustified fears about the use of opioids.

Invasive procedures

Invasive pain treatment procedures are used when the effect of medical treatment is insufficient or in some specific indications.

Anesthetic techniques

Neuroaxial (epidural and spinal) application of opioids. The indication is pain sensitive to opioids, with intolerance to the side effects of systemic application (2-6% of patients). Intraventricular application is also possible here.

Neurolytic blockades (96% ethyl alcohol, 6% phenol, cold physiological solution) are used minimally due to serious adverse effects; they are recommended only for patients in whom it is impossible to control the pain in other ways and the perspective of survival time is short. An exception is early neurolytic blockade of the celiac plexus in the pancreas and upper abdomen tumors.

Neurosurgical - ablation techniques

They are still considered high-risk and, due to severe side effects, are only recommended for patients in whom it is impossible to control pain in other ways, and the perspective time of survival is short. Currently, the incidence of their use is reported in 1-5% of patients with tumor pain.

Treatment of chronic non-cancer pain

A patient with chronic non-tumor pain and pain in diabetic foot syndrome can be most simply characterized as a “3-D PROBLEM”:

1. the patient is Disabled
2. the patient is usually Depressed
3. the patient shows signs of addiction to Drugs

The treatment must be complex, and a multidisciplinary approach is used the most here, where the following principles apply:

a) Eliminate the use of analgesics, especially opioids and sedatives.
b) Protect the patient from further invasive procedures, and teach him self-control of pain and stress.
c) Reduce potential emotional sources of chronic pain, improve mood and sleep, eliminate depression, and maximize the patient's participation and responsibility in pain control.
d) Motivate the patient to increase activity, try to return to work, do housework activities and hobbies, and decrease the patient's disability.

Treatment of chronic non-cancer pain with persistent organic damage is the most difficult. The goal is not to eliminate pain, nor is this usually possible, but physical rehabilitation and/or withdrawal of analgesics. It requires a multidisciplinary approach and should always be consulted and mainly conducted at workplaces specializing in chronic pain treatment. Under no circumstances should these patients be prescribed addictive drugs, including opioids. This indication can only be made after all other options have been exhausted and carefully considered in the chronic pain management facility. Even then, this procedure must be regularly checked and re-evaluated.

Pain treatment - algesiology

It was approved (Gazette of Ministry of Health of Slovakia. No. 15 dated 9/10/1998, 46, p. 136-137) as an additional medical field above the basic clinical fields of anesthesiology and intensive care medicine, internal medicine, pediatrics, and neurology.

The medical field fulfills the following goals:

- Treatment of chronic pain syndromes that cannot be treated at the required professional level in everyday practice.
- Timely diagnosis and effective treatment of cancer pain to the extent corresponding to the stage of the disease (diagnosis, progression, terminal stage) so that it is available to all oncology patients (hospitalized, outpatient, and at home).
- Treatment of selected acute pain syndromes that require an interdisciplinary approach, thereby ensuring the prevention of chronic pain.

- Improving the quality and availability of acute pain treatment - in the form of a conciliar service for acute pain, specially designed for postoperative, post-traumatic, and obstetrics analgesia.
- Special attention is paid to diagnosing and rationally treating acute, chronic, and tumor pain in neonatology and pediatrics.
- Participates in preventing and treating excessive use of analgesics and psychoactive substances.

References

Aitkenhead A. R., Smith G.: Textbook of anesthesia. 3rd ed, Churchill Livingstone, 1966, 788 s.

Jacox A., Carr D.B., Payne R., et al. Management of Cancer Pain. Clinical Practice Guideline No. 9. AHCPR Publication No. 94-0592, Rockville, MD. 1994: 257.

Klener P.: Léčba bolesti u nádorových onemocnění. Remedia, 1-2, 1995, 30-34

Kočan L, Martuliak I., Ogurčáková D., Vašková J., Kočanová H. Oxidačný stres u pacientov dlhodobo liečených opiatmi /In: Paliatívna medicína a liečba bolesti. - ISSN 1337-9917. - Roč. 8, supl. 2 (2015), s. 23.

Miloschewski D.: Regionální anestezie. Astra, 1998, 208 s.

Rokyta R.: Bolest, morfologické a fysiologické základy. Remedia, 1-2, 1995, 64-70

Ševčík P. a kol.: Bolest a možnosti její kontroly. IDVPZ, 1994

Striebel, W. H.: Terapia chronických bolestí, Osveta, Martin 1993, s. 131

Venglarčík V, Križanský R, Valky J,, Je v súčasnosti anestéziologickou technikou voľ by v chirurgii hornej končatiny ultrazvukom navádzaná regionálna anestézia – UGRA? Anestéziológia a intenzívna medicína, 2014; 3(1)

Chapter 13

Nursing Care of a Patient with a Diabetic Foot

Zuzana Slezáková, PhD.*

Faculty of Nursing and Professional Health Studies, The Slovak Medical University in Bratislava, Slovakia

Abstract

Nursing care for a patient with a diabetic foot is among the most demanding nursing care as it concerns chronic wounds. The nurse assesses the patient's health status, identifies current and potential factors supporting the formation and development of the wound, and assesses nutritional status, fluid balance, and incontinence. Mobility assessment is also essential. Nursing care for a chronic wound requires regular evaluation of the progress of wound healing. Within the nursing process, nurses determine the patient's needs and problems. Based on this knowledge, nursing diagnoses are determined according to the NANDA-I Taxonomy (North American Association for Nursing Diagnosis International). According to the urgency of nursing diagnoses, goals and especially interventions will be selected with the patient or his relatives, and a nursing plan will be created. The nurse's interventions in it must be closely related to the local treatment of the wound and the treatment of the wound's causes. After being informed by the health workers, follow-up care and shared patient decision-making in the nursing process and home care is also a part of the patient's care. Nursing care should support such decision-making because patients with chronic wounds want to participate in decision-making, care planning, and expected outcomes.

Key Words: nursing care, diabetic foot

---

* Corresponding Author's Email: slezakova63@gmail.com

In: Diabetic Foot
Editor: Martina Zavacká
ISBN: 979-8-89113-019-7

Introduction

Nurses determine the patient's needs and problems as part of the nursing process. Based on this knowledge, according to the NANDA-I (North American Association for Nursing Diagnosis International) classification, the following nursing diagnoses are most often determined in patients with wounds. Goals and main interventions will be determined, and a nursing plan will be created with the patient or his relatives, depending on the urgency. Interventions in this plan must be closely related to the local treatment of the wound and the treatment of the wound's cause.

Nursing care for a patient with a diabetic foot is among the most demanding nursing care as it concerns chronic wounds. The nurse assesses the patient's health status, identifies current and potential factors supporting the formation and development of the wound, and assesses nutritional status, fluid balance, and incontinence. Mobility assessment is also essential.

Nurse interventions

1. The nurse assesses and records the characteristics of the wound: etiology, localization, size (length, width, depth, presence of fistulas,) healing

Table 13.1 The most common nursing problems in a patient with a diabetic foot and chronic wound determined by the nurse

Nursing diagnoses	Code	Domain	Class
Impaired skin integrity	00046	11 Safety/protection	2 Physical damage
Impaired tissue integrity	00044	11 Safety/protection	2 Physical damage
Risk of infection	00004	11 Safety/protection	1 Infections
Acute pain	00132	12 Comfort	1 Body comfort
Chronic pain	00133	12 Comfort	1 Body comfort
Social isolation	00053	12 Comfort	3 Social comfort
Disturbed body image	00118	6 Self-perception	3 Body image
Impaired walking	0008	4 Activity/rest	2 Activity/exercise
Disturbed sleep pattern	00198	4 Activity/rest	1 Sleep/rest
Fear of the prognosis of the disease	00148	9 Load handling/tolerance	2 Responses to load handling
Inefficient care for one's health	00078	1 Health support	2 Health Management

phase, the surrounding area of the wound base, secretion (amount, color, odor). A mnemonic can be used: MEASURE).
MEASURE

M = (measure) dimensions of the wound (length, width, depth, and area),
E = (exudate) exudate (quantity and quality),
A = (appearance) appearance (wound bed, including type and amount of tissue),
S = (suffering) suffering (type and level of pain),
U = (undermining) undermining (presence or absence),
R = (reevaluate) reevaluation (regular monitoring of all parameters)
E = (edge) edge (state of the edge of the wound and the surrounding skin).

The skin, wound, or bandage odor should be recorded. When applying/changing the dressing and cleaning the wound bed, gently remove the dressing in the direction of hair growth. If necessary, clean the wound with normal saline solution or the prescribed solution and gently dry it with gauze. Apply the dressing to the wound according to the manufacturer's instructions. If necessary, tamp the wound cavity with a dressing (gauze, alginate).

2. The nurse takes a photograph of the wound for documentation purposes. Wound documentation must include data on wound location, etiology, classification, clinical signs, exudate, odor, bleeding, and wound bed. The condition of the surrounding skin, the size of the wound, the depth of the wound, and its length and width are evaluated. Pain is essential for assessing the wound; we consider its localization, intensity, character, and duration. It is crucial to assess the circulation of the peripheral part of the body. The records must include the time of applying/changing the dressing, the therapeutic and cleaning agents used, and the frequency of the dressing change.
3. The nurse takes a specimen from the wound, following the so-called ten recommendations:
   a) The patient should be informed about the specimen collection. The doctor/physician explains to the patient the reason for taking the sample for microbiological examination and describes the procedure.
   b) Before the collection itself, removing all impurities from the wound, such as necrotic tissue, dried exudate, and remnants of covering material, is essential. The wound is cleaned with sterile NaCl 0.9%, Ringer's solution, or by debridement.
   c) Sterile swabs made of cotton or artificial silk on a stick are used for the smear. If the wound is moist, using a sampling tampon directly from the package is possible. If the wound is dry, the swab should be

moistened with sterile NaCl 0.9% or Ringer's solution to increase the probability of collecting microorganisms.

d) The tampon should only come into contact with the wound's surface.
e) We move the tampon on the surface of the wound using the so-called ten points technique, and at the same time, we use the "zig-zag" method. With light pressure, we roll the tampon and turn it 360 °. Light pressure on the wound causes gradation of the patient's pain.
f) The specimen should be taken from a representative wound area. In cases of extensive wounds, we collect using several tampons in different places (which show the most significant signs of infection, changed color and consistency, and the presence of exudate) from the bed and the edges of the wound.
g) We place the swab in the transport medium, label it, and arrange its delivery to the laboratory.
h) We fill out the application and remember to write down the location of the wound, the place of collection, and the type of antibiotics the patient uses.
i) Specimens should be transported to the laboratory as quickly as possible and processed optimally within 4 hours after collection.
j) The laboratory result contains a list of isolated potential pathogens, their quantity, and antibiotic sensitivity.

4. We monitor the clinical signs of the wound, such as exudate, odor, skin condition, condition of the wound area, signs of inflammation, swelling, redness, or other changes in skin color. We remember to monitor pain using pain intensity rating scales. Measuring the wound is an essential part of wound monitoring.
5. Photographic documentation is an integral part of wound monitoring and evaluation. If performed correctly, it gives us the most accurate and up-to-date information about the wound. It is irreplaceable proof of the quality of provided care. The patient's written consent with photo documentation of the wound is not required, but the patient's personality and ethical principles must always be respected. Photo documentation enables all persons involved in wound assessment to find their bearings in the wound, clearly and comprehensibly demonstrate clinical progression, and accurately and correctly record and evaluate the patient's health status. We can motivate and educate the patient after presenting images where improvement is visible. Principles for photo documentation:
   - Take pictures without touching the wound.
   - Always take pictures from the same angle, from the same distance, with the same camera, and with the same zoom.

- Place a label with the patient's name, date, wound number, and a ruler near the wound.
- The label must not touch the wound or damage the area around the wound.
- Save, label, and archive the pictures.

6. The nurse monitors long-term normoglycemia and weight, adherence to diet No. 9. and ensures sipping, i.e., clinical oral administration of nutritional supplements. This continuous sipping of a liquid diet at short intervals throughout the day has proven particularly effective in hospitalized patients who cannot take in sufficient amounts of food. The product, which is intended directly for patients with diabetes, is Diasip in two flavors; it contains important vitamins and trace elements necessary for wound treatment,
7. The nurse is responsible for applying and changing dressings, one of the most crucial parts of diabetic foot syndrome treatment. An adequately made dressing can lead to the defect's faster and more effective healing. However, it is essential to use the right tools and materials. When changing a dressing, it is also necessary to observe the principles of asepsis and proper documentation of the dressing. Follow the dressing change instructions for the nurses:
   - Prepare the patient for the procedure, and help him to take a suitable position.
   - Prepare the aids so that they are easily accessible.
   - Hygienically wash your hands and put on gloves.
   - Check the appearance of the dressing before removing the cover.
   - Remove the dressing and covering, do not damage the base of the wound.
   - Evaluate and record the wound (photo documentation).
   - Remove the remains of ointments and pastes from around the wound, and assess the area around the wound.
   - Rinse the wound with a rinse solution.
   - Depending on the condition of the wound, select a suitable therapeutic cover.
   - Treat the surrounding wound area.
   - Apply the primary coverage chosen in advance.
   - Overlay the primary coverage with the secondary coverage.
   - Depending on the doctor's instructions, apply a fixation cover using a short-stretch bandage.
   - After the dressing is finished, help the patient to take the original position

- Take care of cleaning the tools.
- Wash and disinfect your hands.
- Make the record of wound evaluation and dressing to the documentation.
- Dressing must be performed under aseptic conditions.
- During the entire procedure, communicate with the patient.

8. Record the wound in the patient's file according to the following recommended criteria:
   - types of wounds and classification of the severity of the wound
   - diabetic foot ulcer: Wagner-Armstrong classification
   - previous diagnostic and therapeutic interventions and their effects.
   - Localization of the wound: graphically, in writing, and possibly also photographically
   - Duration of wound
   - Number of relapses
   - Wound size: greatest length (cm), greatest width (cm) 90° to length, depth (cm), wound pocketing, fistulas, undermining: determine the place using clock position (head represents 12 o'clock/legs 6 o'clock)
   - Wound base / most common tissue types:
     - granulation tissue,
     - fibrin tissue,
     - moist or dry avital tissue,
     - dermis,
     - adipose tissue,
     - muscle, fascia,
     - tendon,
     - bone.
   - Exudate–quantity: none, little, much
   - quality: e.g., cloudy, serous, bloody.
   - Wound odor: yes/no
   - Wound edges: e.g., flat, convex, undermined, vital, macerated, hyperkeratotic
   - Surroundings of the wound: e.g., redness, swelling, blister, maceration, dry/ moist skin
   - Signs of inflammation
   - Pain in or near the wound.

   It is important to record these basic criteria of wound assessment depending on technical possibilities and practicability, either on paper or in electronic form, and to provide photographs. In addition, it is also advisable to record whether the patient understands the cause of the wound and the time course of wound treatment, what limitations he has based on the treatment, what aids he has, and how he can take care of himself, or with his relatives to help treat the wound and manage everyday situations.

9. The nurse follows the principles of moist wound healing and covering:
   a) When choosing the right cover, it is necessary to respect the phases of wound healing (hemostatic, inflammatory, granulation, epithelization, remodeling). When there are several phases of wound healing, a cover whose properties are most suitable for the dominant phase of wound healing should be chosen. The size of the primary cover must be selected so that the entire wound is in contact with the functional part of the cover; the possible overlap beyond the edges of the wound respects the manufacturer's instructions.
   b) In the case of a deeper and undermined wound, choosing a packing of primary coverage) is necessary (prevention of empty spaces in the wound.
   c) The size of the secondary cover should be chosen so that the edges of the cover exceed each edge of the wound by at least 2 cm.
   d) The composite and adhesive covering size should be chosen so that the entire wound is in contact with the active part of the covering, which fulfills the function of the primary coverage. The overlap of the wound's edges with the active part respects the manufacturer's instructions.
   e) Minimizing the number of dressing changes while maintaining constant adequate moisture and temperature in the wound is necessary.
   f) Adequately choose the coverage according to the amount of exudate and secretion (prevention of leakage, maceration of the wound and its edges, and prevention of drying of the wound).
   g) Ensuring an atraumatic dressing (preventing tearing of the newly formed tissue).
10. The nurse regularly checks, compares, and records every change,
11. The nurse positions the affected body part.
12. The nurse educates the patient and family members about the wound care procedure.
13. The nurse applies analgesics according to the doctor's prescription and monitors their analgesic effect.
14. The nurse informs the patient that most defects are caused by imperfect foot care and wearing inappropriate shoes. Patients are advised:
    - Not to use sharp objects for pedicures
    - Not to cut their own nails with bad eyesight

- Not to take hot baths, not to use thermofor or other electrical appliances
- Not to sit near the fire
- Not to walk barefoot, not even at home
- Not to wear shoes with a high heel and a narrow tip.

Recommendations for patients:

- Inspect the feet and area between the toes daily; if the patients cannot do it themselves, someone else must check it.
- Wash your feet when necessary, take a daily foot bath, possibly with antifungal solutions, and dry areas between your toes. Well-dried feet, even in the intermediate layers, should be lubricated with a thin layer of easily absorbed cream.
- Cut your nails immediately after soaking them in lukewarm water.
- Avoid walking barefoot.
- Chemical and special plasters and pumice stones must be used to remove the calloused, hard skin.
- Check the shoes from the inside as well. Before putting the shoes on, it is necessary to make sure that there is no foreign body (most often a stone) in the shoes.
- Patients with poor vision should not treat feet and nails (the help of a loved one).
- Daily self-examination focused on possible new rhagades or blisters. Use a mirror or ask a family member for help. Up to 71% of people with diabetes with limb complications simultaneously have poor vision and impaired mobility and cannot check their legs by themselves!
- Use cream for dry skin.
- Change your socks daily, preferably light-colored, without rubber bands or garters. Never walk without socks.
- Do not wear stockings with a seam.
- Cut the nails straight, and inform the pedicurist about the diabetes diagnosis.
- Pathological lesions on the legs or any injury should be reported to a medical professional.
- Strengthen the interdigital muscles with leg and toe exercises.
- Take off your shoes at the doctor's office. Some studies show that if a person with diabetes is barefoot during an outpatient examination, the doctor will check his feet in 65-72% of the cases, but if he comes with shoes on, the foot check is only 12-19%.
- Check bruises, hyperkeratosis, blisters, fungi, onychomycosis, rhagades, and skin color and temperature changes. It is necessary to assess further deformities, such as hammertoes, hallux valgus

(bunions), foot arch, osteoarthropathy, and cheiroarthropathy. At least once a year, performing auscultation of arteries, palpation of peripheral pulsations, and non-invasive Doppler examination of vessels, including color mapping, is necessary.

Contemporary, suitable dressing materials and wound dressings

In clinical practice, various dressing materials are used to cover wounds, which are recommended and selected according to the cause and stage of wound healing. We briefly describe their purpose and effects.

Alginates: they have an autolytic effect; they can absorb a small amount of wound exudate and form a gel; they are hemostatic due to their calcium content. They have a bacteriostatic effect and excellent absorption capacity. Secondary coverage is necessary for alginates. They are indicated for exuding plaque, contaminated, infected wounds, decubitus, and crural ulcers. It is not suitable for dry wounds. They are ideal for infected wound edges. They need a secondary cover. Change every 2-3 days. The products are, e.g., Suprasorb A, Melgisorb, Askina Sorb, Sorbalgon, SeaSorb Soft, Kaltostat, and others.

Hydrofibres: Wound exudate is absorbed in only one direction, vertically and not horizontally, providing adequate protection against maceration of the wound edges. It should be placed at least 3-4 cm beyond the edge of the wound.

Hydrocolloids: have a hydroactive and occlusive effect. The size of the hydrocolloid dressing must exceed the wound or the primary dressing below it by at least 3-4 cm on all edges. It is contraindicated for infected wounds. Hydrocolloids stimulate granulation tissue formation and support autolytic debridement, fibrinolysis, and angiogenesis. They are intended for granulating wounds without signs of infection and epithelizing wounds with mild and moderate secretion. Gel is formed on the wound's surface in contact with the exudate. Infected wounds are a contraindication. When used correctly, the coverage must extend beyond the ulcer area. Replacement after 3-5 days. The products are, e.g., Granuflex, Askina Hydro, Hydrocoll, Suprasorb, Comfeel Plus, Adaptic, and others.

Superabsorbents consist of superabsorbent plastic granulate in a plastic or non-woven cover and are used for wounds with very strong exudation. Foil covering: consists of a thin, transparent polyurethane membrane with a polyacrylate adhesive surface. They cannot absorb liquids. They can be used for superficial, non-exuding, epithelizing, and dry wounds.

Medical honey: thanks to its strong osmotic effect, it can actively maintain a moist wound environment by removing lymph and blood plasma from the wound area. Depending on the composition, it has a bacteriostatic to bactericidal effect.

Hydrogels: due to their water content, they rehydrate dry necroses and plaques as part of autolytic debridement, and in this process, fibrin plaques are also released. Enriched hydrogels can have an antiseptic, absorbent, or another different component. Hydrogel representatives are, e.g., Nu-gel, Flamigel, Granugel, Hydrosorb, and others. It is combined with other types of dressings (Tender Wet active cavity, Atrauman Ag, Actisorb Plus, Silvercel). The frequency of dressing changes depends on the condition of the surrounding skin. Covering the gel with a primary and secondary covering, such as a transparent film dressing, is advisable.

Silver bandages: elemental, nanocrystalline, or ionic silver is in various synthetic dressing materials. It has an antibacterial and fungicidal effect and partially neutralizes the smell. They are used for a short time. Activated charcoal dressings: bind odors, and they are used for strongly smelling, infected, and plagued wounds.

Foam bandages: are polyurethane foams rich in pores, which absorb exudate from the wound with the help of capillary force (on average, max. 15-20 ml at 10 x 10 cm); however, this exudate can be rereleased under pressure, and there is a risk of maceration.

Hydropolymers are polyurethane foams that expand upon absorption of exudate and expand towards the wound bed. Depending on the additives (e.g., superabsorbent made of polyacrylate), the exudate may bind in the wound dressing. For sensitive skin, it is also available as a gently adhering foam, e.g., based on silicone.

Negative pressure wound therapy - NPWT cleans the wound and enhances the growth of granulation tissue. It is used, e.g., in dressing the wound bed, treating fistulas, managing infection and exudate, and fixing skin grafts. It belongs to the physical methods of treating open wounds and skin defects. The basic principle of wound therapy with controlled negative pressure is the local effect of sub-atmospheric pressure on the tissues that form the base of the wound. Controlled negative pressure improves debridement and promotes wound healing. The impact of treatment by controlled negative pressure consists of drainage of interstitial fluid, reduced local edema, and increased local blood flow. Thanks to this action, there is a significant suppression of bacterial colonization of the wound, further to mechanical deformation of cells and subsequent cell proliferation. The final effect is an increase in granulation and promotion of epithelization. When using NPWT, there will be a significant reduction in the area of the wound, less pain, and a shorter treatment time. One of the pressure-controlled treatment techniques is the patented VAC. A foam with communicating pores and a drain with side holes are inserted into the wound. The entire wound and the surrounding area are then covered with a film that does not allow the wound to communicate with the surrounding air. The drain is connected to a source of negative pressure, and the secretion from the wound is removed by foam to the drain and from there to the holding reservoir.

Biological debridement with larvae – Maggot therapy, the so-called "biosurgery." Larvae of the common green bottle fly (Lucilia sericata) are grown in sterile conditions. These larvae release proteolytic enzymes and feed mainly on avital tissue.

Cotton, polyester, and viscose are used as a secondary covering for slightly and moderately secreting wounds; they can be used as a primary covering for low-adherent contact layers with the wound or as a secondary covering.

Antiseptic dressings are used in the prophylaxis and therapy of local infection because they are infused with an antibacterial substance. They need secondary coverage. They protect granulation tissue and allow free passage of exudate (Inadine, Betadine ointment).

Antiseptic cover with silver has an antimicrobial effect and contains the active substance ionized Ag^{+} or inert Ag^{0} silver atoms. Silver is also effective against antibiotic-resistant strains such as MRSA. The dressing is used for a critically colonized and clinically infected wound. The products are, e.g., Askina Calgitrol Ag. Contraindication is hypersensitivity to any component of the cover.

Silicones are slightly adherent to the skin. The advantage is that a secondary cover is not necessary. They are flexible to the contours of the body and allow sterile application. They can be in a spray form or sheets. The products are e.g., N - A Ultra, Mepilex, and Askina Silnet.

Bandages with activated carbon and silver–the activated carbon absorbs microorganisms, and silver destroys bacteria absorbed by carbon with its antibacterial effects. They are used for strongly secreting and smelly wounds (Actisorb).

Application of stem cells– this method is the subject of clinical studies. Indications in diabetic foot syndrome are clinical signs of limb ischemia and/or ulceration, gangrene, imminent amputation, and non-healing amputation wound. At the same time, ischemia must be proven by non-invasive vascular examination, and the condition cannot be solved using standard revascularization procedures (PTA, bypass). This method's safety, efficacy, and optimal indication need verification in randomized, controlled, and long-term studies.

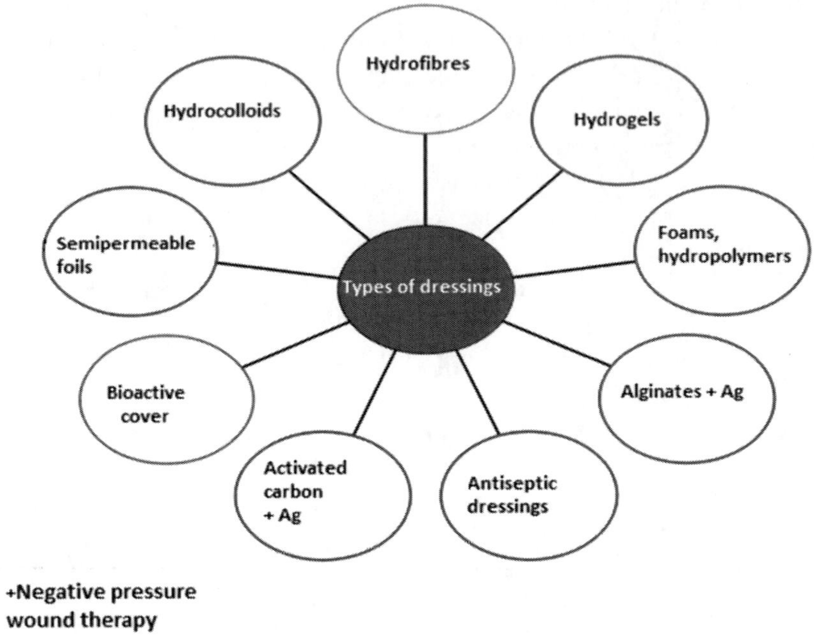

Figure 13.1 Types of dressings.

Hyperbaric oxygen therapy (HBO) involves inhaling oxygen at increased atmospheric pressure (2.5 - 3 times). This leads to an increased partial pressure of oxygen and its physical dissolution in the plasma. Problematic and difficult-to-heal wounds are among the indications for HBO.

Cleaning the wound

Wound cleaning involves the removal of necrotic tissue, fibrin plaque, and other unwanted components in the wound (debridement). On the microscopic level, during debridement, we must consider the presence of biofilm in the wound. Biofilm does not have to be macroscopically visible; it must be expected (stagnation of healing, excessive secretion, presence of typical bacteria, stopping of healing despite local treatment, etc.). Biofilm is a mutually cooperating system of various bacterial colonies in the produced protective matrix, protecting from external influences. Underestimating the presence of biofilm in the wound and its solution will condemn the treatment and healing of the wound to failure. Prerequisites for local biofilm treatment are antimicrobial solutions, thorough mechanical debridement, and choice of coverings, which contain substances directly acting on the biofilm matrix and antimicrobial additives in the period between two dressings.

Mechanical debridement- unwanted components in the wound are non-selectively removed by rubbing and wiping, e.g., gauze square or another suitable tool. It is used when there is a need for immediate and quick removal of unwanted parts from the wound, for home dressings. It does not require special training. It can be painful and cause more bleeding if handled carelessly. This debridement is painful and inappropriate in some nosological units (pyoderma gangrenous, autoimmune diseases). The use of mechanical debridement in combination with an appropriately chosen antiseptic substance potentiates the effect of this debridement against certain levels of biofilm.

Autolytic debridement. It is used in the period between dressings. It is about using suitable covers, which ensures a suitable microenvironment in the wound, especially by hydration and the possibility of migration of elements, activates the autolytic processes to clean the wound.

Enzymatic debridement is relatively affordable, does not require special equipment, and can be used even in the home environment. It is an enzymatic dissolution of necrosis and plaque in the wound. It is more selective than mechanical debridement and is also less painful. Enzymes, mainly in the ointment form, disrupt the wound's enzymatic bonds of necrosis and plaque. However, the enzymatic cleavage products can irritate the wound and its surroundings. They also interact with some antimicrobial solutions, so special attention should be paid to combining solutions and topical ointments.

Chemical debridement includes the use of substances with a direct effect on the bonds of necrosis and plaque in the wound. Complications and use are the same as for enzymatic debridement. Substances that directly disrupt the bonds in the mucopolysaccharide matrix biofilm (e.g., PHMB) can be considered chemical debridement.

Physical debridement The application of physical methods during debridement is less frequent due to financial requirements and needed equipment. Therefore, it is more common in specialized workplaces. The used techniques are debridement with targeted high-pressure water jets (hydrosurgery), cavitation mechanism for releasing necrosis even from undermined areas using ultrasound waves (20-40 MHz), and radio frequency plasma generators (in addition to debridement, which also has a hemostatic effect).

Biological/larval debridement uses larvae of the common green bottle fly grown in laboratory conditions. It is applied directly to the wound or through the enclosed perforated cover. It is the release of proteolytic enzymes into the wound by larvae that consume the decomposed necrotic tissue. Debridement is performed by applying it to the wound, covering it, and changing it at specific intervals. Patient compliance with larvae, bacterial population (Proteus vulgaris, Pseudomonas aeruginosa), laboratory availability, and experienced medical personnel determine the use of biological debridement in practice.

When choosing the type of debridement, we consider the time constraint (sepsis, symptoms of inflammation), then we choose faster forms of debridement (mechanical, sharp, physical). In case of patient intolerance, in some specific conditions (pyoderma gangrenosum, autoimmune ulcerations, hypocoagulable state, oncological ulcerations in palliative mode), we choose less radical forms (enzymatic, biological, autolytic, or chemical).

Completing the debridement when cleaning the wound requires dressing with an antimicrobial/antiseptic solution. Attention should be paid to the manufacturer's stated exposure time (wounds are not poured at, but a dressing is applied, or a mechanical medical spray pump is used). If the exposure time is not followed, the use of the solution changes to a too-expensive rinsing solution.

Prevention of foot problems and follow-up care

Patients without risk factors who have healthy feet should be given general advice on foot hygiene, nail care, and footwear purchase. Their risk status should be reviewed annually.

Patients with any risk factor should be checked more often and instructed about preventive foot care. High-risk patients should be advised to:

- wash and check the feet daily
- use creams or lotions to prevent dry skin and callus formation
- always have the feet measured when buying shoes
- avoid walking barefoot
- prevent thermal injuries (e.g., from hot water bottles, fires)
- seek medical attention for any leg injury or discomfort, however trivial it may seem
- avoid the temptation to try to self-treat calluses and other disorders.

These simple steps have been shown to reduce the incidence of foot ulcers significantly.

The foot tends to lie "between specialties," Many centers have developed diabetic foot care teams that may include a diabetologist, surgeon (vascular and/or orthopedic), chiropodist, specialist nurse, and shoemaker. The team's primary role is foot care education, often provided by a chiropodist or podiatry nurse. The introduction of multidisciplinary teamwork in the community and education of at-risk patients have significantly reduced the number of amputations.

Follow-up care and shared patient decision-making in the nursing process and home care

It is essential to remember that hospitalized patients with diabetes are at potential risk of further insensitive ulceration, mainly if bed rest is prolonged. Protection of the heels and other pressure points is paramount; devices such as leg troughs are invaluable. After discharge, all patients require education about foot care and careful follow-up, preferably by the foot-care team, to prevent recurrent ulceration. Special footwear (e.g., extra-depth shoes with appropriate insoles) is necessary for many patients.

The paradigm of shared decision-making (Shared Decision Making) has emerged in recent years. Sanchez (2019) states that the paradigm incorporates patients' values and preferences concerning a health problem after being informed by health professionals of the possible therapeutic alternatives and expected outcomes, thereby providing patients with an active role in decision-making and care planning. To apply this approach, it is necessary to respect the patient's autonomy, abandon paternalistic models regarding the relationship between health professionals and patients/family members, and respect the principle of patient autonomy. Nursing care should support such decision-making because patients with chronic wounds want to participate. The elements that support this process are closeness and trust, the openness of professionals to the opinions of patients and their families, and personal motivation. Last but not least, positive feelings associated with participation in the decision-making process, such as mental well-being and a sense of productivity also support the process. However, for this process - shared decision-making in home care - there are also barriers, such as:

- older age and especially sensory disorders that come with old age,
- accompanying pathologies such as infections and fever, which prevent them from participating in the decision-making process,
- low level of education in the field of diabetic foot syndrome and therefore do as they are told,
- the impact of a paternalistic model of care organization that prevents them from participating in the treatment of wounds because the doctors decide about the treatment. Patients are very dependent on the professional

competence of doctors. A doctor is like a parent who gives patients the best treatment according to their judgment - this paternalistic approach has been reduced in modern medicine, but not completely.

References

AALAA, M., O. T. MALAZY, M. SANJARI, M. PEIMANI a MR MOHAJERI-TEHRANI. Nurses' role in diabetic foot prevention and care; a review. Journal of Diabetes & Metabolic Disorders [online]. 2012, 11(1) [cit. 2021-6-27]. ISSN 2251-6581. Dostupné z: https://pubmed.ncbi.nlm.nih.gov/23497582

BAŠKOVÁ, M. Podtlaková terapie u novorozence. Léčba ran. 2020, 7(4), 11-12. ISSN 2336- 520X.

DIMUNOVÁ L, RÓNAYOVÁ I, GREŠŠ HALÁSZ B et al. Analysis of chronic wound management in nursing. CSWHI 2020; 11 (3): 65–70. doi 10.22359/cswhi_11_3_10.

FEJFAROVÁ, Vladimíra, JIRKOVSKÁ, Alexandra a kolektiv. Léčba syndromu diabetické nohy odlehčením. 1.vyd. Praha: Maxdorf Jessenius, 2015. 351 s. ISBN 978-80-7345-436-4

GRAY D, WHITE RJ, COOPER P. TRENDS IN WOUND CARE. Vol II. British Journal of Community Nursing monograph. The wound healing continuum. London: Quay Books Division, MA Healthcare Ltd; 2003. 3, 128 p.

GRAY J.E., ENOCH, S., HARDING, K, G. WOUND Assessment. British Medical Journal 2006, no 332, p.285-288.eSSN 156-1833.

HERDMAN T.H., KAMITSURU S., LOPES C.T. (Ed.) NANDA International, Inc. Nursing Diagnoses. Definitions and Classification. 2021- 2023. New York, Stuttgart, Delhi, Rio de Janeiro, Thieme, 2021, ISBN 9781684204540.

HESS C.T. Clinical Guide to Skin and Wound Care. 7th ed.Philadelphia: Lippincott William αWilkins,2012.624p.ISBN 13:978-1-60913-679-6.

HLINKOVÁ E., NEMCOVÁ J., HUĽO E., BALKOVÁ M., MIERTOVÁ M., POKORNÁ A. Management chronických ran. Praha, Grada, 2019, 224 s. ISBN 978-80-271-0620-2

HOLT, P.: Assessment and management of patients with diabetic foot ulcers. Nursing Standard 2007, vol.27,no.27,p.49-55.eISSN 0029-6570

JIRKOVSKÁ, Alexandra, BÉM, Robert. Praktická podiatrie: základy péče o pacienty se syndromem diabetické nohy. Praha: Maxdorf, 2011, 139 s. Jessenius. ISBN 978-80-7345-245-2.

KOZOŇ,V, ŠPAČEK,F, ; GREŠŠ HALÁSZ,B., HUĽO, E. POKORNÁ,A ET al: Multidisciplinárny štandardný postup: Manažment rán. https://www.standardnepostupy.sk/standardy-manazment-ran/,2021, MZSR

KRISTOVÁ, J., SLEZÁKOVÁ, Z., MIKLOVIČOVÁ, E., BACHRATÁ, Z.:Potreby pacientov s chirurgickým spôsobom liečby, Oše obzor, roč. 18, č. 2, 2021, s. 37-43.

KUDLOVÁ, Pavla. Ošetřovatelská péče v diabetologii. Praha: Grada, 2015, s. 212. ISBN 978-80-247-5367-6.

LEAPER DJ et al. (2012) Int Wound J 9(Suppl 2): 1–19

LIBOVÁ, Ľ. a kol. 2020. Ošetrovateľstvo v chirurgii. Hodnotiace a meracie nástroje. Martin: Vydavateľstvo Osveta, 2020. 140 s. ISBN 9788080634919.

MORBACH,S. Diagnostika, ošetrovanie a prevencia syndromu diabetickej nohy. Bratislava:hartman.Rico, 2001.s.45.53.ISBN 80-238-6801-2.

PAVELOVÁ,Ľ, KRIŠTOFOVÁ, E MESÁROŠOVÁ, J., ZRUBCOVÁ,D., VÖRÖSOVÁ, G., SOLGAJOVÁ,A., BEŤKOVÁ, M: Efekt microdacynu v procese hojenia chronických rán.In: Pomáhajúce profesie, roč. 2, č. 2, 2019, 40-51

POKORNÁ, A.: Úvod do wound managmentu- Příručka pro hojení chronických ran pro studeny nelékařských oborů. MU Brno, 1. vydání, 2012. 126s. ISBN 978-80-2010-6048.

REPKOVÁ, A., KUKLÍNKOVÁ, M.: Diabetes mellitus a výskyt vaskulárnych komplikácií. Oše obzor, roč. 10, č. 1-2, 2013, s. 3-6

Sanchez G.: Introduction to "Intramolecular Hydrogen Bonding 2018", Molecules. 2019 Aug; 24(16): 2858.

SÁNCHEZ, G., JOSÉ J., MARTÍNEZ-VIZCAÍNO V., RODRÍGUEZ-MARTÍN B., Patients' and Caregivers' Conceptualisations of Pressure Ulcers and the Process of Decision-Making in theContext of Home Care. International Journal of Environmental Research and Public Health [online]. 2019.16(15): 19-27. DOI: DOI:10.3390/ijerph16152719.

SHAN, A, J., WOLLAK, C, SHAH.J.BWound Measurement Techniques: Comparing the Use Ruler Method,2D Imaging and 3D Scanner. Journal of the American College of Clinical Wound Specialists 2015,no.5,p.52-57.eISSN 2213-2648.

STRYJA, Jan. Repetitorium hojení ran 2. 2.vyd. Semily: Geum, 2016. 377 s. ISBN 978-80-87969-18-2

SUSSMAN, C., BATES-JENSEN, B.M. Wound care: a collaborative practice manual for physical therapists and nurses. 4th ed. Philadelphia: Lippincott William αWilkins,2012.ISBN:978-60831 -715-8.

TEREKOVÁ V, KUBICOVÁ Ľ, OZOGÁNYOVÁ M. Moderné trendy ošetrovania chronických rán. Ošetrovateľský obzor. 2004;1(1–2):8–11. ISSN 0457-4214

VOWDEN P., COOPER R. A. Ein integrativer Ansatz für das Management von Wundinfektionen. European Wound Management Association (EWMA). Position Document: Management of wound infection. London: MEP Ltd, 2006.

ŽĎÁRSKÁ, J. D., KVAPIL, M: Moderní diabetológia. Vyd. Current media, 2017.208 s. ISBN9788088129196.

Conclusion

Martina Zavacká

Successful treatment and prevention of diabetic foot syndrome depend on a holistic approach in which it is seen as a part of multi-organ impairment. Therefore, the teamwork of several experts is necessary. An internist, a diabetologist, an angiologist, a vascular surgeon, and a surgeon with podiatric training play a vital role in this team. They manage diabetes, prevent and treat comorbidities, cooperate in the diagnosis of malnutrition and nutritional therapy, in early diagnosis and effective treatment of infections. Last but not least, the internist works in cooperation with other experts in treating ischemia of the lower limbs, the appropriate choice of therapy, local therapy, and the prevention of ulcers. The common goal of all involved professionals must be the highest possible recovery rate. Optimal use of financial resources is essential here, and high healing rates should be distinct from non-critical primary amputation, which should be avoided. In addition, the remaining foot should have a sufficient function, and the recurrence rate should be kept as low as possible using proper secondary prevention measures. In addition, patient education has also been shown to be essential in delaying the onset or recurrence of diabetic foot ulcers. This includes providing information on basic foot care advice, advice on appropriate footwear, and wound care. A survey to evaluate the effectiveness of patient education on diabetic foot care demonstrated a positive impact on patients' health beliefs, as evidenced by a statistically significant positive change in weight, body mass index, and blood pressure.

Care for a patient with diabetic foot syndrome is often complex. Multidisciplinary and multi-professional teamwork is essential to meet these complex requirements. In addition, interprofessional and intersectoral medical collaboration is vital, as is the integration of non-medical health professionals (diabetes counselor/dietary assistant, pedicurist, orthopedic cobbler). Successful communication between all professional groups and consistent implementation of all defined processes will be critical for this shared care strategy. In addition, it is necessary to create collaborative interfaces between all professional groups for effective patient care.

Index

S

T

U

V

X